Understanding AIDS & HIV

Series Editor: Cara Acred

Volume 243

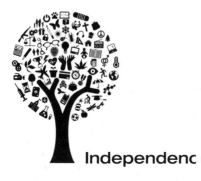

Independence educational Publishers

First published by Independence Educational Publishers

The Studio, High Green

Great Shelford

Cambridge CB22 5EG

England

© Independence 2013

British Library Cataloguing in Publication Data

Understanding AIDS & HIV. -- (Issues ; 243)

1. AIDS (Disease)

I. Series II. Acred, Cara editor of compilation.

616.9'792-dc23

ISBN-13: 978 1 86168 645 9

Printed in Great Britain

MWL Print Group Ltd

Contents

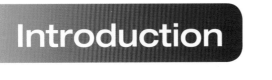

Understanding AIDS & HIV is Volume 243 in the **ISSUES** series. The aim of the series is to offer current, diverse information about important issues in our world, from a UK perspective.

ABOUT UNDERSTANDING AIDS & HIV

Today, everyone has heard of AIDS and HIV. Our understanding of these illnesses is far greater than it ever has been in the past. We know that sexuality and promiscuity do not dictate infection, and we are now challenging the stigma that accompanies a positive test result. In addition to these social breakthroughs, scientific advancements have been hailed as signalling a cure for HIV, and there are continued efforts around the world to reach 'the beginning of the end' of AIDS. Understanding AIDS & HIV explores these issues, and more.

OUR SOURCES

Titles in the **ISSUES** series are designed to function as educational resource books, providing a balanced overview of a specific subject.

The information in our books is comprised of facts, articles and opinions from many different sources, including:

- Newspaper reports and opinion pieces

- Website factsheets

- Magazine and journal articles

- Statistics and surveys

- Government reports

- Literature from special interest groups

A NOTE ON CRITICAL EVALUATION

Because the information reprinted here is from a number of different sources, readers should bear in mind the origin of the text and whether the source is likely to have a particular bias when presenting information (or when conducting their research). It is hoped that, as you read about the many aspects of the issues explored in this book, you will critically evaluate the information presented.

It is important that you decide whether you are being presented with facts or opinions. Does the writer give a biased or unbiased report? If an opinion is being expressed, do you agree with the writer? Is there potential bias to the 'facts' or statistics behind an article?

ASSIGNMENTS

In the back of this book, you will find a selection of assignments designed to help you engage with the articles you have been reading and to explore your own opinions. Some tasks will take longer than others and there is a mixture of design, writing and research based activities that you can complete alone or in a group.

FURTHER RESEARCH

At the end of each article we have listed its source and a website that you can visit if you would like to conduct your own research. Please remember to critically evaluate any sources that you consult and consider whether the information you are viewing is accurate and unbiased.

AIDS and HIV

HIV is a virus which is most commonly passed on by sexual contact. HIV attacks cells of the immune system. Untreated, the immune system weakens so that the body cannot defend against various bacteria, viruses and other germs. This is when AIDS (commonly now called late-stage HIV infection) develops. However, early detection and treatment with antiretroviral therapy (ART) means that people living with HIV can lead active, healthy lives, although they may get side-effects from the treatment.

What are HIV and AIDS?

HIV stands for human immunodeficiency virus. This is a virus in the group of viruses called retroviruses. HIV destroys cells in the body called CD4 T cells. CD4 T cells are a type of lymphocyte (a white blood cell). These are important cells involved in protecting the body against various bacteria, viruses and other germs. HIV actually multiplies within CD4 cells. HIV cannot be destroyed by white blood cells, as it keeps on changing its outer coat, so protecting itself.

AIDS stands for acquired immunodeficiency syndrome. This is a term which covers the range of infections and illnesses which can result from a weakened immune system caused by HIV. Because ART has altered the way we think about the condition, the term late-stage HIV is being increasingly used instead of AIDS.

Note: HIV and AIDS are not the same thing and people who get HIV infection do not automatically develop AIDS. AIDS is unlikely to develop in people who have been treated in the early stages of HIV infection. Even in people who do not receive treatment, there is usually a time lag of several years between first being infected with HIV and then developing infections and other AIDS-related problems. This is because it usually takes several years for the number of CD4 T cells to reduce to a level where your immune system is weakened.

People with HIV can pass the virus on to others whether or not they have any symptoms.

How do you become infected with HIV?

⇨ **Sexual transmission.** This is the most common way to pass the virus on. In 2010, it accounted for about 19 in 20 new confirmed cases in the UK. Semen, vaginal secretions and blood from an infected person contain HIV. The virus can enter the body through the lining of the vagina, vulva, penis, rectum or mouth during sex. Having vaginal or anal sex with an infected person is the most common route. Oral sex carries a much lower risk but this can increase if you have a condition which affects the defence barriers of the mouth, such as ulcers, bleeding or damaged gums or a sore throat. You cannot be infected with HIV by coming into contact with the saliva of an infected person (for example, through kissing or coming into contact with spit). HIV is not passed on by coughing or sneezing.

⇨ **Needle sharing.** HIV (and other viruses such as hepatitis B and hepatitis C) can be passed on by people who are dependent on injectable drugs and share needles, syringes and other injecting equipment which is contaminated with infected blood. However, needle-exchange services run by hospital, clinics and drug dependency units and the more ready availability of medicines taken by mouth (such as methadone) have drastically reduced needle-sharing as a source of infection.

⇨ **Infected blood.** In the past, quite a number of cases occurred from infected blood transfusions and other blood products. This is now rare in the UK, as since 1985 all blood products are checked for HIV before being used. It is still a significant problem in developing countries.

⇨ **Accidental needlestick injuries.** There have been no cases of HIV infection from needlestick injuries in a healthcare setting in the UK since 1999. HIV infection from a needlestick injury outside of a healthcare setting has never been recorded anywhere in the world.

⇨ **From mother to child.** HIV can be passed to an unborn child from an HIV-positive mother. However, with appropriate treatment the risk of transmission of HIV from mother to baby can be reduced to less than one in 100. This means that, with appropriate treatment, the vast majority of babies born to HIV-positive mothers will not have HIV. Achieving this depends on detecting HIV before pregnancy, or, in early pregnancy, when anti-medicines can be taken by the mother. Having a Caesarean section to deliver the baby reduces the risk even further. HIV can occasionally be passed to babies through breast milk during breast-feeding. If formula milk is available, mothers with HIV are encouraged not to breast-feed.

Note: to become infected with HIV, some infected blood, semen or vaginal secretions would have to get into your body. You cannot catch HIV from ordinary contact with someone with HIV, such as hugging, shaking hands or touching, or from sharing food, towels, utensils, swimming pools or telephones.

How common is HIV?

The number of new people diagnosed with HIV in the UK peaked at 8,000 in 2006 and dropped to 6,660 in 2010. The total number of people living with HIV in the UK in 2010 was 91,500. Of these, about nine in 20 resulted from men having sex with men and about nine in 20 were due to heterosexual sex. HIV infection is much more common in many other countries in the world.

How does HIV cause problems in the body?

Once HIV is in your body the virus attaches to and gets into the CD4 T cells. The virus then uses the DNA (the genetic code inside the cell) to replicate (make copies of itself). As new virus particles break out of a CD4 T cell, the cell dies. The new virus particles then attach and enter new CD4 T cells and so the process continues. Millions of new virus particles are made in CD4 T cells each day and millions of CD4 T cells die each day.

To counter the virus destruction the body continues to make new CD4 T cells each day. However, over time, the virus usually wins and the number of CD4 T cells gradually falls (usually over several years). Once the level of CD4 T cells goes below a certain level, your immune system is weakened. If your immune system is severely weakened by HIV infection then you are likely to develop various opportunistic infections. These are infections caused by germs which are commonly around us. You would not normally develop infections from these germs if you have a healthy immune system. A low level of CD4 T cells also increases the risk of developing other conditions which the immune system helps to prevent such as certain cancers.

What are the symptoms of HIV and AIDS?

Primary infection with HIV

When you first become infected with HIV it is known as the primary infection. About eight in ten people develop symptoms at this time. The three most common symptoms (sometimes known as the classic triad) are sore throat, fever and a blotchy red rash. Other symptoms can include feeling sick, diarrhoea, swollen glands, headache, tiredness and general aches and pains. The symptoms can last up to three weeks and are often just thought of as flu or a mild viral illness.

After the primary infection

After any primary infection settles, you can remain without any symptoms for several years. Early testing and treatment has revolutionised our concept of HIV infection, which is now considered a long-term disease (see 'What is the prognosis (outlook)?', below). Even without treatment, there are often no symptoms for a long time (often up to ten years) and many people do not realise that they are even infected. However, the virus continues to multiply, the number of CD4 T cells tends to gradually fall and you can pass on the virus to others. During this time some people with HIV who are otherwise well may develop persistent swollen lymph glands (persistent generalised lymphadenopathy) or night sweats.

In time you may start to develop problems such as recurring mouth ulcers, recurring herpes or shingles infections, or seborrhoeic dermatitis (a skin condition caused by a yeast). Old tuberculosis (TB) infection may reactivate in some cases even before AIDS develops, especially in people in the developing world. Other symptoms of HIV that may occur before AIDS develops include diarrhoea, skin rashes, tiredness and loss of weight.

Symptoms of AIDS

The term AIDS is used to describe the most advanced stages of HIV infection and is being overtaken by the term late-stage HIV. People who are treated early in an HIV infection do not develop this stage. AIDS is a general term which includes various diseases which can result from a very weakened immune system. Typically, a person with AIDS has:

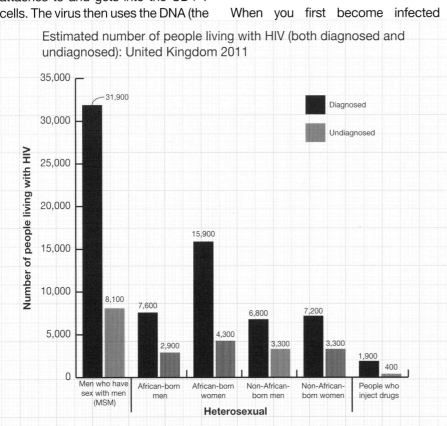

Estimated number of people living with HIV (both diagnosed and undiagnosed): United Kingdom 2011

Source: HIV in the United Kingdom: 2012 Report, November 2012 ©Health Protection Agency

⇨ A very low level of CD4 T cells (around 200 cells per cubic millimetre of blood or below), and/or

⇨ One or more opportunistic infections such as Pneumocystis jirovecii pneumonia, severe thrush in the vagina or mouth, fungal infections, TB, Mycobacterium avium complex, toxoplasmosis, cytomegalovirus, etc. These infections can cause a range of symptoms including sweats, fever, cough, diarrhoea, weight loss and generally feeling unwell.

In addition, people with AIDS have an increased risk of developing other conditions such as:

⇨ Certain cancers. Kaposi's sarcoma is a cancer which is usually only seen in people with AIDS. There is also an increased risk of developing cancer of the cervix and lymphoma.

⇨ An AIDS-related brain illness such as HIV encephalopathy (AIDS dementia).

⇨ A severe body wasting syndrome.

Many different symptoms can develop from the above conditions. Children with AIDS can develop the same opportunistic infections and problems as adults. In addition, they may also develop severe common infections of childhood such as severe ear infections or severe tonsillitis.

What tests are done?

Most sexual health clinics offer a rapid blood test for HIV and can give results within 30 minutes. Even if rapid testing is not available, the results are usually back within a week. Modern tests will pick up the infection a month after first being infected (as opposed to three months with the older tests). GPs can also arrange blood tests but the result will go on your health record. It is recommended that all gay and bisexual men should be tested every year, more often if they have anal sex without a condom, multiple partners, have been diagnosed with another sexually transmitted disease or

develop symptoms of primary or late-stage HIV.

Assessing the extent of disease

If you are confirmed to have HIV then your doctor may do a blood test to check the amount of virus in your blood (the viral load) and the number of CD4 T cells in your blood. These tests may be done from time to time to assess how far the disease has progressed (and the response to treatment).

Tests to diagnose AIDS-related conditions

There is no test for AIDS but you may have a range of other tests to detect opportunistic infections or other AIDS-related conditions. These will depend on the type of symptoms that you develop.

What is the treatment for HIV infection?

Although there is still no cure for HIV, treatment is now effective at allowing people with HIV to live their lives as normally as possible. Since the introduction of medicines to treat HIV, the death rates from AIDS has reduced dramatically. With effective treatment, very few people go on to develop AIDS.

It is not uncommon for people with HIV to feel low or even depressed, especially soon after the diagnosis is made. If you have any feelings of depression then you should speak to your doctor.

Treatment to tackle the virus itself

HIV is now a treatable medical condition and most people with the virus remain fit and well on treatment. Since the 1990s a number of medicines have been developed called antiretroviral medicines. Antiretroviral medicines work against HIV infection by slowing down the replication of the virus in the body. Newer medicines are more effective than medicines used in the past. There are several classes of these medicines which include: nucleoside reverse transcriptase inhibitors (NRTIs), nucleotide reverse transcriptase inhibitors (NtRTIs), protease inhibitors (PIs) and non-nucleoside reverse transcriptase

inhibitors (NNRTIs). Newer classes of medicines have recently been introduced which are integrase inhibitors, fusion inhibitors and CCR5 antagonists. The medicines in each class work in different ways but all work to stop the HIV from replicating itself. This method of treatment is called antiretroviral therapy (ART). You may still occasionally see this referred to as highly active antiretroviral therapy or HAART.

There is a growing body of evidence that taking ART reduces the risk of passing the HIV infection on to others.

Taking three or more antiretroviral medicines at the same time, each attacking HIV at different points in its cycle of replication, is more effective than one or two medicines alone. Taking a combination of different medicines also reduces the risk that the virus will become resistant to any individual medicine. In 2008 the first one pill a day treatment was launched. Each pill contains three different medicines. This is popular, as it is convenient to take and has few side-effects.

The choice of medicines is considered and chosen for each individual patient. The treatment for HIV can be complicated but the majority of people diagnosed with HIV now take antiretroviral treatment in a combination-format just once or twice a day. A team of healthcare professionals is usually involved in looking after you and giving you your treatment.

The aim of treatment is to reduce the viral load to low levels. In most people who are treated with ART, the viral load reduces to very low levels and the number of CD4 T cells rises. This means your immune system is no longer as weakened and you are not likely to develop opportunistic infections. However, it is vital to take the medication regularly and exactly as prescribed to maintain success, and to help to prevent the virus from becoming resistant to the medicines.

As with other powerful medicines, antiretroviral medicines can cause side-effects in some cases. In addition, some of these medicines can react with other commonly used medications. It may be necessary to change an initial combination of medicines to a different combination because of problems with side-effects, reactions or resistance of the virus to an initial medicine. Therefore, different people with HIV can often take different combinations of medicines. Common side-effects include nausea, vomiting and headaches.

When is treatment with antiretroviral medicines started?

As a general rule, antiretroviral medicines are usually started if:

⇨ Your CD4 T cells fall below a certain level (around 350 cells per cubic millimetre of blood or less), even without symptoms. The exact level when treatment is started depends on various factors which your doctor will discuss with you. These include any symptoms present and the rate of decline of the CD4 T cells.

⇨ Opportunistic infections or other AIDS-related problems develop.

However, the treatment of HIV is a rapidly changing area of medicine. Trials are underway to assess whether antiretroviral medicines should be started earlier in people who have no symptoms, even as early as when first infected with HIV. The trials aim to show whether there are benefits from treatment before symptoms develop, which outweigh the risk of side-effects from the medicines. You are likely to have regular blood tests to monitor for side-effects whilst taking treatment.

Treatment and prevention of infections

Wearing a condom when having sex is very important to protect against other sexually transmitted infections, including herpes and hepatitis. People with HIV are usually vaccinated against hepatitis A and hepatitis B, influenza and the pneumococcus (a common cause of pneumonia).

Opportunistic infections are usually treated with antibiotics, antifungals or anti-TB medicines, obviously depending on which infection develops. Even if you have not developed an infection, once the CD4 T cells fall to a low level, you will normally be advised to take a regular dose of one or more antibiotics or other medicines to prevent certain opportunistic infections from developing.

How can infection with HIV be prevented?

There is no vaccine to prevent HIV. Development of one is proving to be very difficult, as the HIV virus is constantly mutating and changing. Therefore, the main way to prevent infection by HIV is to avoid activities that put you at risk, such as sharing needles and having sex without a condom.

Some cases of HIV can be prevented in other ways, for example:

If you are an injecting drug user then do not share needles or other injecting equipment. If available, use local needle exchange schemes.

If you think you have been exposed to HIV through sharing needles or sexual contact you should contact your GP or a sexual health clinic as soon as possible. If it is thought that there is a high risk that you may pick up the infection you will be offered a course of anti-HIV medicines. These are most effective when taken as soon as possible after exposure and certainly within 72 hours.

Healthcare workers should follow local guidelines to reduce the chance of needlestick injury. If you do have an injury, see your occupational health specialist urgently. A course of anti-HIV medicines started as soon as possible and no later than 72 hours after the injury may prevent infection with HIV developing.

If you are pregnant and have HIV infection then you need special antenatal care to reduce the risk of passing on the virus to your baby. HIV treatments can be taken during pregnancy. An HIV test is offered to all pregnant women in the UK.

What is the prognosis (outlook)?

People with HIV who are diagnosed in good time can expect to lead a near-normal lifespan. A study to predict the life-expectancy of men infected with HIV at 30 years of age in 2010 found that they could expect to live to 75, based on access to current treatments. Those who are diagnosed late (with a CD4 count below 350 – the point at which treatment should commence), are more likely to have a poor prognosis. However, even when someone has been diagnosed with a low CD4 count, treatment can effectively bring them back to a good level of health. Life expectancy also depends on other factors such as smoking, alcohol intake and use of other medicines.

In short, for people who have access to modern medicines, the outlook (prognosis) has improved greatly in recent years.

Further help and information

HIV aware

Web: www.hivaware.org.uk

Developed by NAT, the website provides all the basic facts about HIV plus additional information and real stories from people living with HIV.

National Aids Trust

New City Cloisters, 196 Old Street, London, EC1V 9FR

Tel: 020 7814 6767 Web: www.nat.org.uk

Aims to promote a wider understanding of HIV and AIDS, develop and support efforts to prevent the spread of HIV and improve the quality of life of people affected by HIV and AIDS.

Terrence Higgins Trust

314–320 Grays Inn Road, London, WC1X 8DP and various offices around the country (see website)

Tel: 0808 802 1221 for an adviser or 020 7812 1600 for switchboard Web: www.tht.org.uk

A national HIV and sexual health charity. Their helpline offers information and support to anyone living with HIV, affected by HIV indirectly or concerned about their sexual health.

Averting AIDS and HIV (AVERT)

Web: www.avert.org

An international HIV and AIDS charity with lots of useful information on its website.

Tel: 01403 210202 or email info@avert.org

HIV in the United Kingdom

Key findings from the 2012 report by the Health Protection Agency.

⇨ An estimated 96,000 (90,800–102,500) people were living with HIV in the UK by the end of 2011, an increase from 91,500 (85,400–99,000) in 2010. The overall prevalence in 2011 was 1.5 per 1,000 population with the highest rates reported among men who have sex with men (MSM) (47 per 1,000) and the black African community (37 per 1,000).

⇨ 24% (19%–28%) of people living with HIV were unaware of their infection in 2011, the same proportion as seen in 2010.

⇨ In 2011, 6,280 people were newly diagnosed with HIV in the UK, a 21% decline from the peak in new diagnoses in 2005. The decrease is largely due to a reduction in the number of diagnoses reported among those born outside of the UK.

⇨ New diagnoses among MSM have been increasing since 2007 with 3,010 reports in 2011, representing an all-time high. Direct and indirect measures of incidence show that the rate of HIV transmission in this population remains high.

⇨ Over half of the 2,990 heterosexual men and women diagnosed in 2011 probably acquired their HIV infection in the UK, compared to 27% in 2002.

⇨ Rates of new HIV diagnoses and HIV prevalence continue to be significantly higher in London than elsewhere in the UK. The city contains 18 of the 20 local authorities with the highest prevalence of HIV infection.

⇨ Less than 1% of infants born to women diagnosed with HIV prior to delivery acquired perinatal infection in 2010/2011; the overall perinatal transmission rate, for infants born to both diagnosed and undiagnosed women, is estimated to be about 2%.

⇨ There has been a slow but significant decline in the proportion of people diagnosed late (CD4 cell count <350 cells/mm^3) over the past decade, particularly among MSM. Nevertheless, the overall proportion of late diagnoses remained high in 2011 (47%). People diagnosed late have a tenfold increased risk of dying within a year of diagnosis.

⇨ 73,660 people living with a diagnosed HIV infection received care in 2011, representing a 58% increase since 2002. The most deprived areas in the UK also have the highest HIV prevalence; this health inequality is particularly evident in London where diagnosed HIV prevalence is as high as eight per 1,000 in the most deprived areas and less than 1.5 per 1,000 in the least deprived areas.

⇨ 88% of people for whom treatment was indicated were receiving antiretroviral therapy (ART) in 2011. Furthermore, 87% of people receiving HIV care were virally suppressed and were therefore unlikely to be infectious.

⇨ The incidence of tuberculosis (TB) among people diagnosed with HIV has declined over the past decade. Nevertheless, TB incidence among heterosexuals living with diagnosed HIV was substantially greater than that in the general population in 2010. Incidence rates were highest among those diagnosed late and those not on ART.

⇨ In 2011, 70% of all sexually transmitted infection (STI) clinic attendees received an HIV test; with the highest coverage among MSM (83%).

⇨ Almost two-thirds of MSM newly diagnosed as HIV-infected at an STI clinic had not attended that clinic for testing in the previous three years, which strongly suggests there is room for improvement in the frequency of testing by those at highest risk.

⇨ There has been very little commissioning of routine HIV testing of general medical admissions and in the general practice setting.

⇨ In the UK, a trial to investigate the public health effectiveness of pre-exposure prophylaxis (PrEP) in preventing HIV transmission among MSM has begun under the joint leadership of the Medical Research Council Clinical Trials Unit and the Health Protection Agency.

November 2012

⇨ The above information is an extract from *HIV in the United Kingdom: 2012 Report*, and is reprinted with permission from the Health Protection Agency. Please visit www.hpa.org.uk for further information.

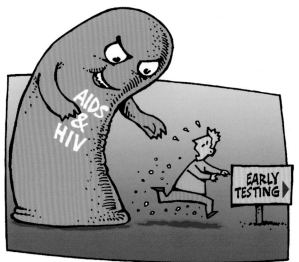

Global facts: World AIDS Day 2012

New HIV infections

⇨ Worldwide, 2.5 million [2.2 million–2.8 million] people became newly infected with HIV in 2011.

⇨ 25 countries have seen a 50% or greater drop in new HIV infections since 2001.

⇨ There has been a 42% reduction in new HIV infections in the Caribbean (the second most affected region in the world after sub-Saharan Africa).

⇨ Half of all reductions in new HIV infections in the last two years have been among newborn children – showing that elimination of new infections in children is possible.

⇨ In 2011, new infections in children were 43% lower than in 2003, and 24% lower than 2009.

⇨ However progress is uneven. Since 2001, the number of people newly infected in the Middle East and North Africa increased by more than 35%. In Eastern Europe and Central Asia, there has also been an increase in new HIV infections in recent years.

AIDS-related deaths

⇨ In 2011, 1.7 million [1.5 million–1.9 million] people died from AIDS-related causes worldwide–24% fewer deaths than in 2005.

⇨ Globally there were more than half a million fewer deaths in 2011 than in 2005.

⇨ The number of AIDS-related deaths declined by nearly one-third in sub-Saharan Africa between 2005 and 2011.

⇨ The Caribbean experienced declines in AIDS-related deaths of 48% between 2005 and 2011 and Oceania 41%.

⇨ However, two regions experienced significant increases in AIDS-related deaths: Eastern Europe and Central Asia (21%) and the Middle East and North Africa (17%).

Antiretroviral therapy

⇨ In 2011, more than eight million people living with HIV had access to antiretroviral therapy.

⇨ The number of people accessing HIV treatment increased by 63% from 2009 to 2011. In ten low- and middle-income countries, more than 80% of those eligible are receiving antiretroviral therapy.

⇨ However, seven million people eligible for HIV treatment still do not have access.

⇨ 72% of children living with HIV who are eligible for treatment do not have access.

People living with HIV

⇨ In 2011, there were 34 million [31.4 million–35.9 million] people living with HIV.

⇨ Sub-Saharan Africa is the region most affected, with nearly one in every 20 adults living with HIV.

⇨ Sub-Saharan Africa accounts for 69% of all people living with HIV.

HIV/TB

⇨ TB-related deaths in people living with HIV have fallen by 25% since 2004.

⇨ However, TB remains the leading cause of death among people living with HIV.

⇨ All people living with both TB and HIV should start antiretroviral therapy immediately as it can reduce the risk of TB illness among people living with HIV by up to 65%.

⇨ However, in 2011, fewer than half (48%) of people with TB who had a documented HIV positive test result obtained antiretroviral therapy.

Women

⇨ Of the 54% of people with access to antiretroviral therapy in low- and middle-income countries, 68% were women.

⇨ Women account for 58% of people living with HIV in sub-Saharan Africa.

⇨ In 26 of 31 countries with generalised epidemics, less than 50% of young women have comprehensive and correct knowledge about HIV.

Key populations

⇨ Among countries with generalised epidemics, HIV prevalence is consistently higher among sex workers in the capital city than in the general population, at around 23%.

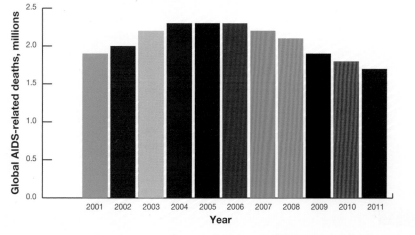

Global AIDS-related deaths 2001–2011

Source: UNAIDS Global Fact Sheet 'World AIDS Day 2012'

- Around three million of the estimated 16 million people who use drugs are living with HIV.

  - In 49 countries with available data, HIV prevalence was 22 times higher in people who use drugs than in the general population.

  - One study suggests that globally, people who inject drugs only use sterile injecting equipment for 5% of injections.

- HIV infection among men who have sex with men in capital cities is on average 13 times higher than in the general population.

- In low- and middle-income countries with available data, 91% of total spending on HIV programmes for sex workers comes from international sources; as does 92% of spending on HIV programmes for men who have sex with men and 92% of spending on HIV programmes for people who inject drugs.

Investments

- US$ 16.8 billion was available from all sources for the AIDS response in 2011.

  - Only a 30% gap in resources remains for fully funding the AIDS response by 2015.

  - The estimated annual need by 2015 is between US$22–24 billion.

- Low- and middle-income countries increased HIV investments by 15% from 2010 to 2011.

  - Domestic public and private spending in low- and middle-income countries rose from US$3.9 billion in 2005 to almost US$8.6 billion in 2011.

20 November 2012

- The above information is reprinted with kind permission from UNAIDS. Please visit www.unaids.org for further information.

Source: UNAIDS Global Fact Sheet 'World AIDS Day 2012'

History of an epidemic

Prior to 1981
HIV transfers to humans in Africa 60–100 years earlier.

1981
First cases of previously unidentified illness reported.

1982
AIDS acronym established for Acquired Immune Deficiency Syndrome.

1983
3,000 cases reported in US of which 1,000 have died.

1984
Scientists in France and US identify HIV as cause of AIDS.

1986
38,000 cases reported from 85 countries.

1990
Eight million people estimated to be living with HIV.

1996
First combination therapy becomes widely available in western countries.

1997
Deaths related to AIDS begin to decline in developed countries and Brazil becomes first developing country to offer universal access to combination therapy.

2002
Botswana begins first national treatment programme in Africa.

2003
Four million people in developing countries are receiving treatment for HIV; however, another 9.5 million are still in immediate need of treatment.

Generic HIV medication becomes more widely available in developing countries.

2006
Estimates show that just 28% of people needing HIV medication in developing countries receive it.

2011
34 million people estimated to be living with HIV worldwide.

Almost half of new HIV infections in the world are among people under 25. Estimates show that more than 7,400 people become infected with HIV daily, 3,300 of whom are young people.

Sources: WHO, USNIH, avert.org

Why are African people and gay men more at risk of HIV?

A lot of work is being carried out to encourage African people and gay men to test for HIV. But why these groups in particular?

By Gavin Williams

The immune system is one of the body's most intelligent designs. By distinguishing between our healthy tissue and infections that aim to attack us, the immune system protects us from diseases and viruses.

So anything that weakens our immune system is a huge, fundamental threat to our health. That is what HIV does. HIV (Human Immunodeficiency Virus) makes it harder for the immune system to fight infection and disease and the final stage of HIV is AIDS, which is when the body can no longer combat life-threatening infections.

Unfortunately, HIV cannot be cured. However, the virus can be controlled and the immune system kept healthy. With the right monitoring and treatment, people with HIV can live a long and normal life. The most important factor in the successful management of HIV is early diagnosis. This is because treatment is far more effective the earlier it is started.

In the UK, over 90,000 people are living with HIV whilst worldwide the number is believed to be around 34 million. People most commonly associate the spread of HIV with sharing needles or by having anal sex. These two activities are very much linked with HIV, but the spread of the virus is not limited to these two things. HIV can be contracted through both anal and vaginal sex. It can also be transmitted through breastfeeding or during pregnancy if the mother is HIV positive.

Each year, the first of December is dedicated to supporting the fight against AIDS and this year marks the first week-long campaign to encourage people to get tested for HIV. Although much progress has been made over the past few decades, there is still a great need to increase awareness of HIV, improve education and fight the prejudice faced by people living with the virus.

It is important to clarify that HIV is not a virus assigned only to specific groups; anyone could contract HIV and anyone – whether hetero or homosexual – is at risk if they don't practise safe sex. Despite this, there are two specific groups that the Terrence Higgins Trust are aiming their HIV Testing Week at. Gay men and African people.

These two groups are more at risk of HIV and it is important to consider why this is the case.

Homosexual men

Gay men have a high risk of contracting HIV; in 2010 the Health Protection Agency estimated that one in 20 gay men in the UK live with HIV, while the ratio is one in 11 in London. Meanwhile, one in 20 gay men in London have undiagnosed HIV.

The increased risk of HIV in gay men can be put down to a combination of lifestyle, physical and cultural factors.

Traditionally, it has been believed that gay men are more likely to test positive for HIV because of their lifestyle; namely because as a group, statistically speaking, gay men are more likely to have more partners, take recreational drugs and have sex without protection.

But these lifestyle factors are surely themselves a product of wider cultural factors. Stonewall suggest that some younger gay men may feel uncomfortable buying extra strong or thick condoms to use for anal sex, as doing so may be viewed as an inadvertent coming out. Moreover, sex education – including lessons on safe sex – are far less likely to be taught with a focus on gay issues than they are with straight issues in mind. If there is less education about safe gay sex, gay men are feasibly less likely to practise it.

There are also biological reasons behind the high risk of HIV in gay men. For example, *Time* suggests that anal sex is 18 times more likely to spread HIV than vaginal sex is. HIV can be found in semen and the lining of the rectum is thin, meaning the virus could easily spread during anal sex.

The most important ways for gay men to reduce their risk of catching HIV is to routinely practise safe sex and to get a HIV test every 12 months if sexually active.

Three in ten gay and bisexual men have never had an HIV test

1 | 2 | 3 | 4 | 5 | 6 | 7 | 8 | 9 | 10

Testing for HIV is increasingly easy – it can even be done using a saliva sample.

African people

In the western world, the fight against HIV has been centred on educating, increasing condom use, testing and counselling. Unfortunately, many African countries do not have the money or resources for this. Unprotected sex is still extremely widespread, therefore so is HIV. Although Africa makes up only about 14.5% of the world's population, the continent is believed to host around 69% of all people living with HIV. In some African countries, the spread of HIV is so severe that it is believed a third of all adults have the virus.

For people born in Africa and now living in the UK, the rate of HIV infection is about one in 20. As well as having a strong cultural history of HIV, there is evidence to suggest that Africans living in the UK are not being educated about HIV risk well enough. Statistically speaking, diagnosis of HIV in African people in the UK is more likely to happen at a later stage of infection. Which means it is more likely to be fatal.

While authorities and healthcare providers must be careful not to stigmatise certain groups or perpetuate the myth that only African and gay communities are at risk of HIV, there is a need for campaigns that can increase early diagnosis of HIV in African-British communities.

Great steps of progress have been made since HIV emerged in the 1980s. However, there is still much work to be done. If more people can be encouraged to take a HIV test – particularly those at a higher risk – then more people can live a long, happy life with HIV and the spread of the virus can be limited.

29 November 2012

⇨ The above information is reprinted with kind permission from author Gavin Williams of Lloydspharmacy Online Doctor. Please visit www.lloydspharmacy.com/doctor for further information.

Gay and bisexual men's health

Sexual health and HIV.

Despite the focus of the NHS on the sexual health of gay and bisexual men and the acknowledged benefits of early HIV diagnosis and regular testing, many gay and bisexual men have never been tested for sexually transmitted infections or HIV.

Sexually transmitted infections

One in four (26 per cent) gay and bisexual men have never been tested for sexually transmitted infections (STIs).

More than four in five (83 per cent) gay and bisexual men who have never been tested said: 'I don't think I'm at risk'. One in seven (13 per cent) are 'scared' to have a test. One in eleven (nine per cent) said they are 'too busy'.

'I've never had any symptoms and therefore not sought help.' Aaron, 44

'I know I should have one but I've never made the effort.' Tyler, 33

'It is difficult to access STI and HIV testing and face-to-face advice when working. Services are never available at times that can fit around work.' Isaac, 52

'My GP refused to speak with me about my sexual health because I came out to him. He instead ushered me out of his office and told me to contact my local GUM clinic.' Nathan, 20

More than two in five (44 per cent) gay and bisexual men have never discussed STIs with a healthcare professional.

In the last five years, 85 per cent of respondents have had sex with men only, ten per cent have had sex with both men and women, one per cent have had sex with women only and five per cent have not had sex with anyone.

'In school we experienced very little sex education and none of the sex education we did receive mentioned or related to same-sex relationships.' Trevor, 18, Wales

'Health (particularly sexual health) issues start at school. I feel that a lack of gay sex education at school constitutes a negative health experience.' Matt, 25, London

HIV

Even though testing for HIV is a Department of Health priority, because early diagnosis reduces onward transmission and facilitates much better treatment, three in ten (30 per cent) gay and bisexual men have never had an HIV test.

Seven in ten gay and bisexual men who haven't tested said they haven't had a test because they don't think they have put themselves at risk. A third said it is because they have never had any symptoms of HIV infection.

One in four gay and bisexual men who haven't had an HIV test said it's because they've never been offered one. One in seven said it's because they don't know where to get a test.

More than half (54 per cent) of gay and bisexual men have never discussed HIV with a healthcare professional.

These figures do raise grave concerns about the effectiveness with which hundreds of millions of pounds of public money have been spent on HIV awareness and prevention in recent years.

⇨ The above information is from *Gay and Bisexual Men's Health Survey* and is reprinted with kind permission from Stonewall. Please visit www.stonewall.org.uk for further information.

Young people's experiences of HIV and AIDS education

Key Findings from the report.

One in four young people learnt nothing about HIV and AIDS at school

A quarter of young people responding to the Sex Education Forum survey (2011) said that they had not learnt about HIV and AIDS in school. A further 11% could not remember if they had learnt anything.

Young people aged 16 and above were more likely than under-16s to state that they had not learnt about HIV and AIDS in school (28% and 19%, respectively). This is promising as it suggests that schools have increased provision – with young people in school today more likely to have learnt about HIV and AIDS than their older peers. Young people educated outside of England were less likely to have learnt about HIV and AIDS than their England-educated peers – 41% of this small cohort answered 'no' they had not learnt about HIV and AIDS in school. However, cohort comparisons within the sample require further research as the sample sizes are small and there may be other factors affecting responses such as differences in how people perceive or remember their education at different ages.

These figures reveal a worrying gap in current provision. Learning about HIV and AIDS and other sexually transmitted disease is the only aspect of sex education that is compulsory for all maintained secondary schools[1]. Sexually transmitted infections are also part of National Curriculum Science for Key Stage 3 but HIV and AIDS are not specifically mentioned.

1   Statutory Instrument 1999 No. 2257 EDUCATION, ENGLAND AND WALES
The Education (Non-Maintained Special Schools) (England) Regulations 1999 In exercise of the powers conferred on the Secretary of State by sections 328(6), 339, 342(2), (4), (5) and (6), 568(5) and 569(4) of the Education Act 1996, the Secretary of State for Education and Employment hereby makes the following regulations: Sex education 11. - (1) Arrangements shall be made to secure that every pupil who is provided with secondary education will receive sex education, or will be wholly or partly excused from such education (except in so far as it is comprised in the National Curriculum) if his parent so requests. (2) The governing body shall, in relation to pupils who are provided with secondary education at the school (a) make and keep up to date a separate written statement of their policy with regard to sex education, and (b) make copies of the statement available for inspection, at all reasonable times, by parents of pupils at the school and provide a copy of the statement free of charge to any such parent who asks for one.
(3) In this Schedule, 'sex education' includes education about-
(a) Acquired Immune Deficiency Syndrome and Human Immunodeficiency Virus, and
(b) any other sexually transmitted disease.

Gaps in knowledge about HIV and AIDS

The survey also asked young people if they had learnt all that they needed to about HIV and AIDS in school. Almost half (49%) answered 'no'. A further 23% were 'unsure' leaving only 28% answering with a definite 'yes'. The younger cohort (aged 11–15) was more likely to give a positive answer with 38% answering 'yes – I learnt all that I needed to about HIV and AIDS in school'. This is encouraging given that some of these young people have not yet completed their schooling.

Further detail was requested about what exactly learning about HIV and AIDS had covered. Young people were most likely to have learnt about the transmission (73%) of HIV and slightly less likely to have learnt about prevention (70%). Learning about stigma and attitudes (41%) and positive living (37%) was less common.

Amongst the younger cohort (11–15 years old) figures were the same for transmission and prevention – but learning about stigma and attitudes (46%) and positive living (44%) was slightly more common than for the older cohort.

The gap in learning about the social aspects of HIV and AIDS reinforces findings from earlier surveys showing that the social and relationship aspects of SRE are too often neglected. Only 21% of young people reported having been taught about skills for coping with relationships compared with 92% who had learnt about the biological aspects of sex and reproduction.

Beyond the four options provided, young people were invited to describe what else they had learnt about. Responses included global issues, getting test results, the symptoms, how it affects your immune system and treatment. Worryingly some young people reported learning incorrect

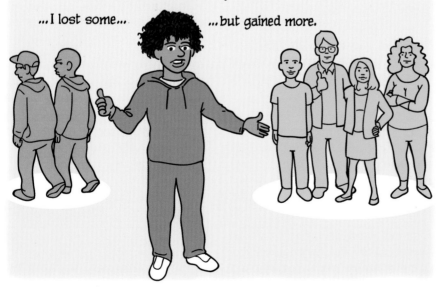

When I came out as HIV positive...
...I lost some... ...but gained more.

information such as 'we were told by our teacher that you could catch AIDS by sitting on a toilet seat that someone with HIV/AIDS had sat on'.

Some respondents took this opportunity to explain that they had only learnt about HIV and AIDS in biology and that SRE had been absent or minimal:

'We went into depth in an AS biology lesson but nothing has been mentioned about the stigma attached or any of the more important emotional side of it.'

'We've barely had any Sex Education at all, and HIV/AIDS hasn't even been mentioned.'

'We didn't cover HIV at all in my memory. If we did it may have been as a passing comment in a science class instead.'

Learning outside school

'I have not been taught anything at school. My mum talked to me about it.'

Young people were asked if they had ever discussed HIV and AIDS with other people, and were asked to pick as many options from the list as they wished. Friends were by far the most common response – almost a quarter of young people had talked about HIV and AIDS with friends (73%). Parent or carer was the second most popular response – a third of young people (33%) ticked this option. Of those young people selecting 'someone else', 11 respondents had spoken to no-one at all. 46 young people had spoken to a teacher, two had spoken to an intimate partner and one had talked about HIV and AIDS within an on-line community.

A question about other information sources showed that the TV (59%) and the Internet (56%) were the most popular sources of information besides school. Young people were invited to tick multiple responses and to specify other sources of information not listed – these included pornography, comic books, the radio, charities and theatre.

May 2011

⇨ The above information is an extract from Young People's Experiences of HIV and AIDS education by Lucy Emmerson. Please visit www.sexeducationforum.org.uk/evidence for further information and a full copy of the report.

© *The Sex Education Forum*

Criminalisation of HIV transmission

The criminal law was first used in the context of HIV transmission in England in 2003 when an individual was found culpable for HIV transmission under the Offences Against the Person Act 1861. Two sections of the act relating to 'grievous bodily harm' can be used to prosecute HIV transmission: Section 18, 'intentional transmission' and Section 20, 'reckless transmission'. However, there has never been a successful prosecution for intentional transmission. Moreover, in England and Wales it is not possible to be charged for 'exposure' where there has been no transmission.

However, the law in Scotland is different. A common law offence of 'culpable and reckless conduct', which may also be called 'causing real injury', is used. Importantly, exposure to a sexually transmitted infection without transmission actually taking place may be a crime in Scotland.

In England and Wales, someone may be guilty of reckless HIV transmission if all five points below applied to them at the time of the alleged offence:

⇨ They knew they had HIV.

⇨ They understood how HIV is transmitted.

⇨ They had sex with someone who did not know they had HIV.

⇨ They had sex without a condom.

⇨ They transmitted HIV to that person.[1]

There is no evidence to suggest that criminalisation will impede the spread of HIV. On the contrary, advocates believe that it contributes to the stigmatisation of people with HIV, undermines the notion that HIV prevention is a responsibility that is shared between HIV-negative and HIV-positive people, and discourages people from testing for HIV.

Internationally, such laws are often applied selectively, targeting particularly marginalised groups.[2] In the UK, many of the first cases were prosecutions of black African men. However, since then, a wider variety of individuals with HIV have been prosecuted.

References

1. Bernard EJ *Transmission of HIV as a criminal offence.* in Social and legal issues for people with HIV, NAM, 2010

2. Jürgens R et al. *Ten reasons to oppose the criminalisation of HIV exposure or transmission.* Reproductive Health Matters 17: 163–172, 2009

⇨ The above information is reprinted with kind permission from NAM Publications. Please visit www.aidsmap.com for further information.

© *NAM Publications 2013*

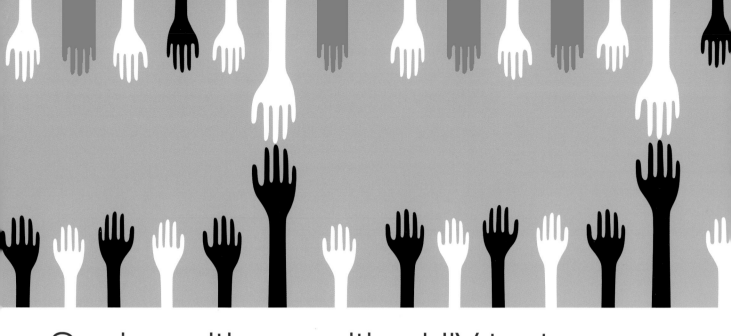

Coping with a positive HIV test

Hearing that your HIV test is positive can be shocking, but many people with HIV live a long and healthy life. Find out how to cope with a positive test result and where to go for support if you need it.

There's no right or wrong way to feel when you test positive for HIV, but there are things you can do to help you cope with the result

Angela Reynolds of the Terrence Higgins Trust (THT) says it's important to remember that HIV treatments have improved. This means HIV is now a manageable long-term condition. 'If you're tested early and get appropriate healthcare and treatment, your life expectancy is normal,' she says.

Your emotions

You may feel a range of emotions when you get your test results. This could include shock, numbness, denial, anger, sadness and frustration. It's perfectly normal and understandable to feel any of these. 'Some people might also feel relief that they finally know the truth,' says Reynolds.

You may also feel isolated and alone, even if you have family and friends around you. Whatever you feel, you don't have to go through it alone, and there are ways you can help yourself cope better.

Getting the test result

You will usually be given your results in person. The doctor, nurse or health adviser will do another HIV test to confirm the result, assess your current health and refer you to specialist HIV services. They will also talk to you about how you feel and help you think about where you can get support.

'They may ask you what your plans are for the next few days, who is at home for you, and where you are going to go after this appointment,' says Reynolds. 'They will also give you details of organisations you can contact if you want to.'

The doctor, nurse or health adviser will also talk about safer sex and the importance of using a condom for vaginal, anal and oral sex to avoid passing on the virus to a sexual partner.

As part of the discussion about safer sex, the doctor or nurse may discuss how you can change your behaviour to prevent passing the virus on. Find out more about preventing transmission of HIV.

Getting up-to-date information

'It's not unusual to feel shocked and unable to take everything in,' says Reynolds. 'Don't feel you have to remember everything in one go. You should be given written information, and you can always ask questions of your medical team or a helpline.'

Find out as much as you can about HIV, its treatments and side-effects. 'Talk to health professionals and use reliable websites,' says Reynolds. 'This will dispel any myths you hear about HIV. It will also help you understand the information you are told about your condition, and help you ask the right questions of the team who provide your care.'

Don't rely on information you've heard in the past or which may be out of date. Make sure the information you have is accurate. Up-to-date, accurate information is available from national services such as THT, your local HIV services and HIV information from NHS Choices.

Learning to cope

Accepting that you're HIV positive can be the first step in getting on with your life. 'Be honest with yourself,' advises Reynolds. 'You will have this for the rest of your life. But remember that although HIV is not curable, it is treatable.'

You might imagine that you'll be ill all the time and will have to stop

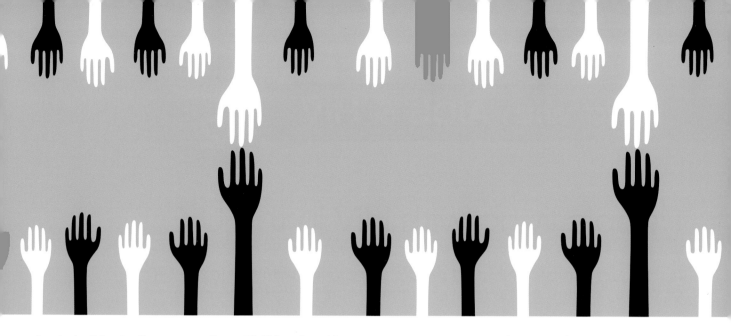

work, but this isn't necessarily the case. 'Most people carry on working and don't have to give up sex and relationships forever,' says Reynolds. 'After the first shock of diagnosis, most people cope over time. There's a lot of support to help you.'

Try not to keep your feelings to yourself. If you don't feel you can talk to friends or family, try talking to your doctor, nurse or a counsellor, or call a helpline. Find counselling services near you.

Websites such as namlife and healthtalkonline can guide you through the first few weeks and months after your diagnosis. They can also give you an insight into how other people have coped with an HIV diagnosis and how it has affected their lives.

Your strengths

Reynolds suggests learning from a time in the past when you dealt with a difficult situation. 'Everyone has different ways of coping,' she says. 'If you look back at how you have coped in the past, you might be able to identify what helped you cope before. This can give you confidence that you'll be able to cope with this new situation. If you feel you could have coped better, think what you could do differently now. For example, if you didn't talk to anyone the last time you had a problem in your life, you could talk to a health adviser this time. Work out in advance what your coping strategy will be.'

Talking to others

Talking about what you're going through can help, but think carefully about who you tell about your diagnosis.

'Try and stay in control of who you disclose your health status to,' suggests Reynolds. 'Don't rush into telling anyone. Work out why you want to tell them and think of the potential consequences, for example if they tell someone else. If you decide to tell them, work out how you will answer any questions they might ask, such as 'How did you get it?''

If your family or partner would like support to help them cope with your diagnosis, they can also contact HIV organisations.

As well as talking to a doctor, nurse, friends or family about how you're feeling, you might also want to meet other people with HIV. Finding out how other people have coped with a positive diagnosis, and hearing about their experiences of living with HIV, can be helpful for some people. There are support groups for people who have recently found out they're HIV positive. Your GP, HIV clinic or a helpline can let you know what's available in your area.

There are also support groups for specific people, such as young people, women, gay people, people from Africa and people who are HIV negative and have a partner who is HIV positive.

The website healthtalkonline has videos and articles about people's

experiences of living with HIV, including getting an HIV diagnosis.

If you're feeling depressed

It's normal to feel as though you're not coping at times, to stop enjoying being with friends and family, or to feel sad or have trouble sleeping. However, if these feelings last a long time or you continue to feel overwhelmed by them, you may have depression. Get help as soon as possible as you may need treatment. Your GP, HIV clinic or local mental health services can all help you.

Diagnosis during pregnancy

Pregnant women in the UK are offered an HIV test as part of routine antenatal care. Finding out you're HIV positive when you're pregnant can be very difficult for you and your partner. Your midwife and HIV services will support you and help reduce the risk to your baby. It's possible to give birth to a healthy baby who is HIV negative. Find out more about HIV, pregnancy and women's health on the i-Base website.

9 November 2012

⇨ The above information is reprinted with kind permission from NHS Choices. Please visit www.nhs.uk for further information.

© *NHS Choices 2012*

People living with HIV in the UK

In 2011, an estimated 96,000 people were living with HIV in the UK. Of these, around a quarter were unaware of their HIV infection.

The overall proportion of people living with HIV in the UK was estimated to be 0.15%, or one in 650. The proportion of men living with HIV in the UK was estimated to be 0.20%, or one in 500, while the proportion of women living with HIV in the UK was estimated to be 0.09% or one in 1,000.

This information is based on the Health Protection Agency's calculations for 2011 as seen in their *HIV in the United Kingdom: 2012 Report*.

How many people have been diagnosed and are receiving HIV specialist care?

In 2011 there were 73,659 people in the UK living with a diagnosed HIV infection and receiving care.

How has this been changing over time?

The number of people receiving HIV specialist care has increased every year in the last decade, from 30,849 in 2002 to 73,659 in 2011. This is a 58% increase.

What about people of different genders?

About two thirds of people receiving HIV specialist care were male.

This information is based on the Health Protection Agency's figures for the numbers of HIV positive people who were receiving HIV care in the UK in 2011: 49,083 males, and 24,576 females, as seen in the HPA's *HIV in the United Kingdom: 2012 Report*.

What about people in different probable exposure categories?

Of those living with HIV in the UK and receiving HIV specialist care, more people were infected through sex between men than through heterosexual sex. A large proportion of those living with diagnosed HIV in the UK infected through heterosexual sex were infected outside the UK, whilst most of the men who have sex with men living with HIV in the UK acquired their infection within the UK.

Of those receiving HIV care in 2011, 36,355 were exposed through sex between a man and a woman, 31,825 were exposed through sex between men, 1,636 were exposed from injecting drug use, 1,488 were exposed from mother-to-child transmission and 533 were exposed from blood/receiving blood products.

What about people of different ethnicities?

Over half of people receiving HIV specialist care in the UK were white, and over a third were black African.

What about people of different ages?

Two-thirds of all people living with a diagnosed HIV infection in 2011 were aged between 30 and 49, but there are significant numbers both of young people and older people now living with HIV.

What about people in the different nations of the UK?

The vast majority of people receiving

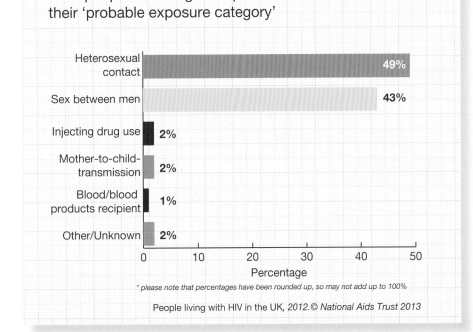

% of people receiving HIV specialist care in the UK and their 'probable exposure category'

Category	Percentage
Heterosexual contact	49%
Sex between men	43%
Injecting drug use	2%
Mother-to-child-transmission	2%
Blood/blood products recipient	1%
Other/Unknown	2%

Percentage

* please note that percentages have been rounded up, so may not add up to 100%

People living with HIV in the UK, 2012.© National Aids Trust 2013

HIV care in the UK were living in England.

What about people in the different regions within England?

42% of people living with HIV in the UK in 2011 were living in London. This is a slight increase from 2010 (43%).

Figures range from 31,147 in London and 6,766 in the North West to 1,385 in the North East and 3,400 in the East Midlands.

⇨ The above information is reprinted with kind permission from National Aids Trust (NAT). Please visit www.nat.org.uk for further information.

Living with HIV in the UK, the facts:

Some people living with HIV in the UK still experience prejudice and discrimination which can be more difficult than living with the physical effects of HIV.

Stigma and discrimination are often the result of ignorance about how HIV is passed on and unfounded fear about becoming infected.

Because of the communities in the UK who are most affected, HIV-related discrimination is often exacerbated by homophobia, racism or negative attitudes towards immigrants and asylum seekers.

People living with HIV report experiencing stigma and discrimination most frequently:

- in the workplace
- in the NHS – particularly amongst healthcare workers who aren't HIV specialists (e.g. GPs and dentists)
- in the media – where reporting of HIV is often inaccurate and misleading and fuels existing prejudices
- amongst family and friends.

Information from the National Aids Trust HIV Factsheet.

What is stigma?

AIDS-related stigma and discrimination means prejudice, negative attitudes, abuse and maltreatment directed at people living with HIV and AIDS. Many people with HIV and AIDS are shunned by family, friends and community. They are treated poorly at the hospital and school. Even at places of worship, worshippers refuse to sit by them.

Stigma towards people living with HIV is very wrong. This is because not everyone had the virus from wrong behaviour. If even they did, we are all human and we all make mistakes. We therefore have to accept them and love them, BUT take care not to engage in any risky behaviour with them.

Factors that contribute to HIV/AIDS-related stigma include:

⇨ HIV/AIDS is a life-threatening disease, and therefore people fear to relate to it.

⇨ HIV infection is associated with behaviours such as homosexuality, drug addiction, prostitution or promiscuity, that are already unaccepted in many societies.

⇨ There is a lot of inaccurate information about how HIV is transmitted, creating irrational behaviour and misperceptions of personal risk.

⇨ HIV infection is often thought to be the result of personal irresponsibility.

⇨ Religious or moral beliefs lead some people to believe that being infected with HIV is the result of

moral fault (such as promiscuity) that deserves to be punished.

⇨ The effects of antiretroviral therapy on people's physical appearance can result in forced disclosure and discrimination based on appearance.

Possible consequences of HIV-related stigma to be:

⇨ Loss of income/livelihood

⇨ Loss of marriage and childbearing options

⇨ Poor care within the health sector

⇨ Withdrawal of care giving in the home

⇨ Loss of hope and feelings of worthlessness

⇨ Loss of reputation.

Stigma towards people living with HIV is very wrong. This is because not everyone had the virus from wrong behaviour. If even they did, we are all human and we all make mistakes. We therefore have to accept them and love them, BUT take care not to engage in any risky behaviour with them.

⇨ The above information is reprinted with kind permission from eSchooltoday. Please visit www.eschooltoday.com for further information.

Stigma and discrimination

The term stigma refers to any attribute that marks an individual as being unacceptably different from other people. Stigmatising attitudes contrast those who are 'normal' with those who are seen as 'abnormal' or 'deviant': they can therefore be seen as part of a process of social control.[1] HIV is not the only medical condition which has been stigmatised (others have included tuberculosis, cancer, depression and other mental health issues).

Within black African communities, pejorative understandings of people with HIV are often linked to perceptions of their sexual behaviour (promiscuity, prostitution, homosexuality, etc.) as well as to fears that the infection is readily transmissible. Moreover, HIV infection may be seen as a 'death sentence', in the light of previous experiences in African countries when treatments were not available.[2, 3]

HIV stigma results in HIV being perceived as an issue that affects 'other people' and makes informed discussion of the topic difficult. As such, it contributes to the onward transmission of HIV and low rates of testing in black African communities as well as affecting the life of people with diagnosed HIV.

There are a number of different ways of describing and categorising stigma. One approach[4] distinguishes:

Enacted stigma: actual experience of discriminatory acts.

Anticipated stigma: fear of such discrimination, which may lead to concealment.

Internalised stigma (self-stigma): the person accepts the negative social attitudes as valid.

In a series of qualitative research studies [3, 5, 6, 7, 8, 9] black African people with HIV have reported instances of enacted stigma after they have disclosed their HIV status or when others have realised they have HIV. Individuals have been asked to leave shared accommodation by relatives or by housemates. Others have found that due to irrational fears of contamination, people avoided all physical contact with them, prevented children from playing with them, were concerned about shared use of bathrooms, and kept items such as cups and cutlery separate.

Awareness of a person's HIV status can lead others to question the person's sexual morality, which threatens their role in the family and the wider community. Individuals may be cut off from their partner and kept away from their children. When the information has reached relatives 'back home' in Africa, these relationships have also been profoundly altered, sometimes affecting key sources of social support.

Faith groups and leaders, usually a very important source of support,

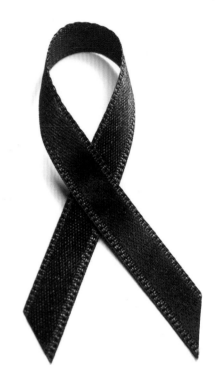

have on occasion asked individuals with HIV to leave a congregation or expressed hostility to antiretroviral treatments.[5, 8]

Although much of the enacted stigma comes from within black African communities, it also occurs from wider society. In employment, individuals may be discriminated against because of their HIV status or experience breaches of confidentiality. In antenatal and other healthcare settings, individuals have reported distressing treatment and overwhelming ignorance regarding infection control procedures from some staff. Moreover, press coverage which portrays black Africans in the UK as bringing infection into the country and burdening the NHS is often experienced as stigmatising. Similarly, press coverage of criminal prosecutions for HIV transmission has been stigmatising.

As noted above, stigma may also be 'anticipated': in other words, the person with HIV is concerned about stigmatisation that may happen, or afraid of it. As a result, they do not disclose their HIV status and avoid circumstances where stigma may be encountered. These strategies greatly reduce the experience

1 Parker R and Aggelton P *HIV and AIDS-related stigma and discrimination: a conceptual framework and implications for action*. Social Science and Medicine 57: 13-24, 2003

2 Flowers P et al. *Diagnosis and stigma and identity amongst HIV positive Black Africans living in the UK*. Psychology and Health 21: 109-122, 2006

3 Burns F et al. *Why the(y) wait? Key informant understandings of factors contributing to late presentation and poor utilization of HIV health and social care services by African migrants in Britain*. AIDS Care, 19: 102-108, 2007

4 Weiss MG *Stigma and the social burden of neglected tropical diseases*. PLOS Neglected Tropical Diseases 2: e237, 2008

5 Doyal L, Anderson J *'My fear is to fall in love again...' how HIV-positive African women survive in London*. Social Science and Medicine 60:1729–1738, 2005

6 Doyal L et al. *'I want to survive, I want to win, I want tomorrow': An exploratory study of African men living with HIV in London*. Homerton University Hospital NHS Foundation Trust/Terrence Higgins Trust, September 2005

7 Dodds C. et al. *Outsider status: Stigma and discrimination experienced by Gay men and African people with HIV*. Sigma Research, 2004

8 Doyal L et al. *'You are not yourself': exploring masculinities among heterosexual African men living with HIV in London*. Social Science and Medicine 68:1901-1907, 2009

9 Doyal L et al. *My Heart is Loaded: African Women Surviving With HIV in London*. The Health Foundation/Terrence Higgins Trust, 2003

AIDS & HIV: The regional picture

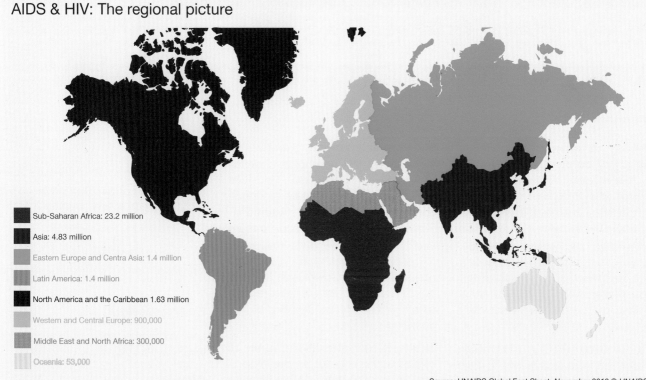

Sub-Saharan Africa: 23.2 million

Asia: 4.83 million

Eastern Europe and Centra Asia: 1.4 million

Latin America: 1.4 million

North America and the Caribbean 1.63 million

Western and Central Europe: 900,000

Middle East and North Africa: 300,000

Oceania: 53,000

Source: UNAIDS Global Fact Sheet, *November 2012 © UNAIDS*

of enacted stigma. Nonetheless, sometimes individuals may anticipate stigma to be worse than it actually would be in reality.

A study with black African women found that for many, controlling information about their HIV status represented the single most important challenge in their daily lives.[5] The fear of negative reactions to disclosure of this information and concerns about losing control over how far the news would spread have been widely reported in a number of studies. Moreover, this frequently leads to a weakening of key relationships, depletion of a person's social life, isolation, and prevents individuals from getting social support. Black African people may already feel excluded from the majority population because of their differing ethnic background, but HIV can also exclude them from their own community.[10, 2, 5, 8, 3]

Specifically in terms of dealing with HIV, the danger of accidental disclosure can discourage individuals from storing their medication in shared accommodation, taking medication in front of others, taking medication generally, because it is thought to lead to visible side-effects, or going to HIV treatment and support services.

Because of fear of violence, verbal abuse and abandonment, some women do not disclose to their sexual partners.[5] Similarly, black African men who have sex with men are particularly reluctant to disclose their status because they might be blamed for bringing their infection upon themselves, because of their sexuality.[10]

People may also avoid disclosing their HIV status at work, making it harder to manage periods of ill-health or other issues. Linked to this, one study found that people took jobs they were overqualified for.[10]

The third form of stigma is internalised stigma (or 'self-stigmatisation'). Here, the person with HIV comes to share and accept the negative evaluation of him or herself by others.

It is commonly reported that the initial diagnosis of HIV is a great shock. However, in the long term, some individuals are able to come to terms with being HIV positive and live postively. For example, they may be proud of having been able to face up to a challenging situation.

On the other hand, others find it hard to move on from an overwhelmingly

10 Paparini S et al. *'I count myself as being in a different world': African gay and bisexual men living with HIV in London.* An exploratory study. AIDS Care, 20, pp. 601-605, 2008

negative view of the situation and of themselves. They may feel ashamed.

A number of studies report on respondents seeing HIV diagnosis as a death sentence; giving up all hope for the future; giving up on aspirations regarding children, marriage, education, wealth or employment. Some individuals stop caring about what will happen to them, withdraw socially and experience depression. Moreover, in one study it was found that black African men with HIV often used the metaphor of 'weakness' to describe their physical, psychological and economic position. They found it hard to manage their identity as an African man alongside their HIV status.[5, 8, 2]

Such experiences may be interpreted as being manifestations of internalised stigma.

⇨ The above information is reprinted with kind permission from NAM Publications. Please visit www.aidsmap.com for further information.

© NAM Publications 2013

Study identifies issues affecting the quality of life of patients living with HIV

By Michael Carter

Fears about transmitting HIV to others, worries about the future, self-esteem problems, difficulty sleeping and treatment issues are now important quality of life concerns for people living with HIV that are not measured by existing resources, according to a report on a new quality of life measurement tool published in the online edition of the *Journal of Acquired Immune Deficiency Syndromes*.

The tool – called PROQOL-HIV (Patient Report Outcomes Quality of Life-HIV) – was developed with the participation of 152 HIV-positive patients in nine countries on five continents.

'PROQOL-HIV is a novel multidimensional HIV-specific HRQL [health-related quality of life] instrument that strives to be sensitive to socio-cultural context, disease stage and treatment in the HAART [highly active antiretroviral therapy] era,' write the authors. 'Important new HRQL issues were uncovered from the culturally diverse experiences of PLWHA [people living with HIV/AIDS] in previously under-represented populations.'

Effective antiretroviral therapy has transformed the prognosis of many HIV-positive patients. However, people living with HIV still experience considerable changes in their health-related quality of life. Tools to measure such outcomes were developed in the era before potent HIV treatment became available. Moreover, they did not take account of the geographic, ethnic and cultural diversity of the epidemic.

Therefore, an international team of investigators set out to develop a new instrument that was sensitive to the impact of HIV therapy, different diseases stages and applicable across settings. It derived from in-depth interviews conducted with patients living with HIV in 2007 and 2008. The patients were recruited in high-, middle- and low-income countries.

The interviews identified 11 broad areas of concern.

General health perceptions

In all countries, patients made spontaneous reference to the importance of their general health. Even slight improvements or declines were considered to have an important impact on quality of life.

Social relationships

The quality of relationships with partners, family and friends was identified as being very important to quality of life. This included receiving support from a main partner, feeling socially acceptable despite illness or side-effects, actual and perceived stigma, the fear of transmission of HIV to others, worries over rejection, loneliness and difficulties with disclosure.

Emotions

A wide range of negative self-perceptions and emotions were perceived to affect quality of life. These included feelings of shame, guilt, inferiority, inadequacy or embarrassment. Also common were sadness, anxiety, irritability and stress.

Energy/fatigue

Low physical and mental energy levels were commonly reported.

Sleep

Many patients described difficulties falling asleep and reduced sleep time. Pain was a frequent case, as was worry and thinking about the consequences of infection with HIV.

Cognitive function

Problems with memory, attentiveness and forgetfulness were reported by a number of individuals. These difficulties had emerged since infection with HIV or the initiation of antiretroviral therapy.

Physical and daily activities

Participants described having to rest more often and difficulty performing day-to-day tasks such as walking short distances or carrying light objects.

Coping

Individuals who were able to integrate HIV and its treatment into their daily routine generally described themselves as coping well. Religious or spiritual beliefs were also considered beneficial for coping.

The future

Fears about the future because of HIV were reported by large numbers of patients. Difficulties planning for the future were also common. There was a perception that HIV would lead to a deterioration in health and some patients believed that even minor infections such as flu would be fatal.

Symptoms

HIV symptoms and treatment-related side-effects emerged as key quality of life issues.

Treatment

Patients regarded treatment as life-saving. Nevertheless, there were concerns about adherence and some patients in low- and middle-income countries feared that supplies of medicines would dry up.

The investigators noted that a number of key quality of health concerns were not covered by existing questionnaires. These include fear of infecting others, concerns for the future, satisfaction with care, self-esteem problems, conception and raising a family, sleeping difficulties, and the impact of HIV on work.

'We identified 11 HRQL themes that broadly encapsulated the HIV experience. Subsumed within these themes were seven issues important to HIV patients yet absent from any single existing instrument,' comment the authors. 'Incorporation of the newly identified issues into HRQL measurement via PROQOL is clearly a step forward in accounting for the long-term experience of living with HIV in the HAART era.'

They conclude: 'PROQOL-HIV shows much promise as an HRQL instrument reflective of the themes that dominate the experience of HIV patients...and important issues which are not measured by existing instruments. It has been developed simultaneously across nine countries, following rigorous international standards.'

4 January 2012

⇨ The above information is reprinted with kind permission from NAM Publications. Please visit www.aidsmap.com for further information.

HIV survivors: alive, but facing poverty, loneliness and prejudice

Thousands heading into an old age they did not think they would see, having given up jobs expecting to die young.

By Sarah Boseley

In the 1980s and 1990s they were told they were going to die young, so they gave up their jobs and cashed in the pensions they wouldn't need, buried their friends and tried to make the most of their last months on Earth.

Decades later, thousands of men and women with HIV in the UK, US and across the world are heading into an old age they never expected to see. In the US in 2001, 17% of people with HIV were over 50. Now that figure stands at 39% and by 2017 it will be half. In the UK, the Health Protection Agency says one in six people (16.8%) being seen for HIV care in 2008 were over 50 – and that will double in the next five years.

Many of those who were saved by the discovery of antiretroviral drugs in the early 1990s felt it was a miracle to be alive. But life for the survivors of HIV, as they age, is bittersweet. Many are poor and have long since been edged out of the workforce. Half a lifetime spent on powerful drugs has taken its toll. Aside from the physical health issues as a result of the virus, there are high rates of mental health problems too.

John Rock, from Sydney, Australia, was diagnosed with HIV 30 years ago. 'My partner started getting sick in 1983 and died early in 1996,' he said at an international Aids conference in Washington DC. 'Many of my colleagues and friends were pushed out of the workforce around the mid-90s because they were not well enough to work. Subsequently, triple combinations (of antiretroviral drugs) came along

and they are still alive, but at the peak of their earning capacity they were out of the workforce for ten years. Now they are destined for a retirement they thought they never would have, but it's going to be in poverty.'

Lisa Power from the Terrence Higgins Trust (THT), who spoke at the conference about the ageing HIV-positive community in the UK, acknowledged the unfortunate consequences of advice from support groups to those who were thought to be dying. 'In the 1980s and 90s we encouraged people to give up work and go on state benefits and not be economically productive,' she said. 'Now we have condemned people to live on an old-age state pension.'

Money is not the only need. Many feel lonely and isolated. In a video made for a project called *The Graying of HIV* in the US, Bill Rydwels, 77, from Chicago, recalled a time of terror and sadness when AIDS was scything down his friends. It was nonetheless a time of warmth and support that he no longer has. 'It's just so much better today and yet it is a lonelier time. Years ago it was a time that we all spent together. It was a terrible time and a wonderful time because you got to know everybody very, very well. They cried on your shoulder and laughed with you. You don't get that any more.'

Recent research from THT in the UK reveals similar sadness. James, 61, a gay man living in the UK who did not want to give his full name, is suffering from serious health problems, including blindness resulting from the use of an experimental drug to treat another condition (not HIV). 'My life is empty,' he told researchers. 'I have tried so hard over the last ten years to fill the emptiness. Worked really hard at it. I am in a cul-de-sac. It would be nice just to have somebody to telephone.

'I am fed up with people at the top of HIV organisations saying because there is combination therapy everyone is fine. People with neuropathy, and in wheelchairs, we are the forgotten people.'

Half the world away, in Africa, which now bears the brunt of the epidemic, the numbers of older people with HIV are also rising fast. Epidemiologists at the University of Sydney estimate that there are more than three million people over 50 with HIV in sub-Saharan Africa, and that the figure is rising rapidly.

Ruth Waryero, from Kenya, now 65, had an HIV test when she was 48. She went home and told her husband. 'He listened to me and then he got up and said, it's up to you.

'Take care of yourself – I'm off. Since that time I have not seen him again and yet he was the breadwinner in the family. He left me with the four children and two years later I had two grandchildren.

'In Kenya we have different problems [from those in Europe]. Older men try to get younger women for sex. They ignore you because as far as you are concerned, you are finished. You don't need sex and they can apply to the young girls.

'But when you are old you are likely to be raped by those who are positive because they believe if they rape you, as old as you are, they will turn negative.'

Older women can also face embarrassment at clinics when they go for tests or drugs, she said. They are asked who they are collecting the drugs for.

'You are not supposed to have sex at your age,' she said. 'As a woman they ask if you are a sugar mummy. I say this HIV came from an old man and the old man has run away from me.'

The older HIV generation – in Africa and elsewhere – is not only made up of those diagnosed years ago. Some are people who have been diagnosed late, having lived for years without knowing they were infected. And many people are now becoming infected later in life.

Laura, who took part in the THT research, is a white, heterosexual, divorced mother of two. At the age of 52 she started a new relationship and then suddenly became ill. Because her symptoms were similar to those of a friend who had been diagnosed with HIV, she took a test. When she was told it was positive, she felt numbness and shock, she said. She cannot believe, as a well-educated person, that she stopped using condoms with her partner and allowed it to happen.

Mark Brennan-Ing, from the AIDS Community Research Initiative of America, told the conference of the 'fragile social networks among people living with HIV in the US and Europe'. Families have abandoned them or do not give them enough help, meaning they end up relying on friends, who often have HIV themselves.

Men who have sex with men, he said, are much less likely to have partners, spouses or children to care for them in their old age. Many of those interviewed live in fear of encountering hostility and rejection in care homes. A 52-year-old gay man from London told the THT: 'I am somewhat fearful of a lonely old age. In practical terms, if I become mentally or physically frail, the prospect of being the only gay man in an old people's home is very frightening indeed.'

27 July 2012

⇨ The above article originally appeared in *The Guardian* and is reprinted with kind permission. Please visit www.guardian.co.uk for further information.

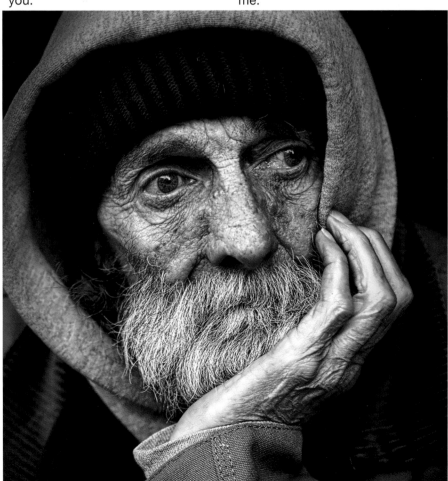

21st Century HIV

Jack's Story

'I'd last had a full sexual health check-up in October 2009. Depending on how 'lucky' I'd been, these check-ups could either be six or 12 months apart, just like a check-up at the dentist. It was the beginning of September 2010, so I booked an appointment at the clinic.

"I just knew – I just knew ... it was the HIV test that had come back positive"

'It was a week after my check-up on a Friday morning when a text came through on my phone telling me there was: 'No need for any follow up appointment.' To be honest, I didn't expect to have anything. When I was younger I had more of a sex drive, now it's a different state of affairs. I forwarded it straight onto my best mate Sven. We're housemates too, and he's always my first port of call with news of any kind.

'I work on public transport and the following Monday, on a morning shift, I was up to my neck in extremely unhappy passengers as we were running late. Customers were screaming at me left, right and centre. In the midst of all this I got a telephone call. The funny thing is I never usually take personal calls at work, it's not like me. A withheld telephone number came up on my mobile and I answered without thinking really. One of the clinic's health advisers was on the end of the line. She told me I needed to come back in to be seen. I told her it must be a mistake and that I'd had an all-clear text sent to my mobile the previous Friday. I imagine she must have been nervous. She said: "No, that had been an error."

'It's funny, I knew – I just knew. Something told me instinctively. I thought there was no other reason why they would call. I asked her which test result was positive and she told me it was the HIV test.

'In the moments afterwards I became surprisingly pragmatic. I was responsible for, I daresay, 900 people on a train, the person accountable for the safety of everyone onboard. The only thing I could think to myself was: 'This will have to be dealt with at 3pm this afternoon when I go to see the health adviser, until then I'll have to put up with it.' I know it sounds cold, but I had to prioritise – I have a job and I needed to get it done. So, moments after finding out I was HIV positive, I carried on working my shift.

'Things didn't run smoothly, ending up with me being delayed at work and having to ring the nurse to tell her I was going to be late. I called Sven to tell him too, so he wasn't wondering where I was. I didn't want to panic him about this, but I didn't want to lie to him over the phone either. When I told him I had to go back to the clinic he asked me why. I said to him: "What would you not want me to have?" and he got it straightaway. He asked me if I was OK and told me he was so sorry. He's really very humane, really compassionate. That's the way he is. Telling him not to worry, that I'd be fine, I said I'd rather know than not know.

'I finally got to the clinic and was called in by the health adviser. She was very apologetic. The person who had sent the text had picked up someone else's file. I could see she was genuinely concerned that this blunder had happened, but what can you do – it was a simple case of human error.

'Later that evening I had arranged to visit an ex-boyfriend of mine after work, but then had to phone him to let him know I'd be later than expected. An hour-and-a-half after I'd seen the health adviser, I picked him up to take him to the supermarket. He told me how selfish I was for being late. I can remember crying with laughter, amazed at how selfish he was being without realising, as I listened to him instruct me to put items of shopping into his trolley.

"My heart goes out to the people who were first diagnosed 30 years ago"

'I'm quite philosophical about the fact that I got HIV from someone else. When you work with the general public, you learn about human beings. We all make mistakes, what's the point of going down a line of retaliation? Everyone has the right to learn, everyone has the possibility to learn from a mistake, from this mistake. Being angry is only destructive in the long run. I'm not angry about how this came about, I can remember as a young man feeling much more vindictive about these kinds of situations. I'm so much happier now to offer others the benefit of the doubt.

'My heart goes out to the people who were first diagnosed 30 years ago, that must have been awful. No one knew anything – imagine the speculation, the fear. Even in the 1990s, it was dreadful for people with HIV. My boyfriend in 1989 was positive, he was a lovely person. Unfortunately he died of AIDS in 1996. The only anti-HIV medication then was AZT which wasn't entirely effective. New combination therapy could have saved him. It's so sad.

'I had a wonderful relationship with a South African boyfriend in 1998 who was also positive. Back then no medication was available to help him in South Africa, no NHS, no Terrence Higgins Trust, not a thing except a placement on a medical trial from one of the big drug companies. He also sadly died a few years later.

"Being angry is only destructive in the long run. I'm not angry about how this came about"

'I'm so lucky, I know what it is to give and be given compassion. Just look at what we have now, it's a first class service with the NHS. And I do really feel lucky. After I was diagnosed I got organised with support, got involved with my local Terrence Higgins Trust service, which has been great. Having one-to-one sessions there with an HIV worker has taught me a lot. I was given good advice, he talked a lot to me about disclosure, when to be cautious and how to approach it.

"I had a wonderful relationship with a South African boyfriend in 1998 who was also positive… he died a few years later"

'I held back from really thinking about HIV until I became more comfortable with it. That probably took a couple of weeks. Since then I've been very proactive about understanding my HIV, so knowing what CD4 counts are, what viral load is – it's mammoth. You need to be careful you don't take on too much and get punch drunk on all the information. I've never been to university and I've only learnt how to use a computer in the last five years. So I got as much information as I could, doing it a bit at a time. Initially I was concerned that I didn't want people to find out my status until I'd got my head around it myself. When you're getting used to something, you can feel vulnerable and in the beginning I felt extremely exposed.

'I found out about a treatment study which was exploring the best time to start antiretroviral therapy. I read up on all the information and it took me about six weeks to make up my mind. There were many issues that came up so I didn't rush into it. There's no point signing up to something if you're not comfortable. I figure that other people have done the same thing in the past in order for us to have drugs now and so I wanted to do something, to have a purpose, a motivation, to help other people and to be of benefit to others in the future. I made an appointment at the teaching hospital to see a research nurse and told them I wanted to go onto the study. I've been on the trial now since the beginning of February. I'm getting on with my life and if I go onto meds, I'll be on meds. If not, then I'm not.

'I'll be volunteering for Terrence Higgins Trust soon and I'm really excited about that. As for work, I've started the ball rolling with disclosing. They don't have an HIV policy yet, but I'm taking them to task as we speak. Each day, I'm learning more and more so, bottom line, I'll be able to help others and that in turn will help me.

'I know who I caught HIV from, but I'm not angry with him. I've come to terms with my diagnosis and it doesn't seem like such an overwhelming issue for me now. That's just how it is. We live in this culture that's revenge mad, some people are hurt and want to feel they've had justice served. I have been lucky enough to always get regular sexual health check-ups, for over 25 years now. Being diagnosed within six months of becoming infected with HIV puts me in the driving seat of my condition. It's given me the opportunity to take control, get good support and make rational decisions about my lifestyle. I've enhanced my diet and exercise when I can, I value each and every day and don't take things for granted. What's the alternative 'car crash' scenario? Having no sexual health check-ups and just carrying on my life in complete ignorance of my positive status until one day HIV was in control of my life?

"I was concerned that I didn't want people to find out my status until I'd got my head around it myself"

'Now I can make plans and be more aware. I can take more responsibility for myself and do much more for other people. There's no such thing as "fair" in life. We may all aspire for things to be fair, but it isn't like that. One of life's gifts is to be able to let things go and then to move on. Being caught in a catch 22 cycle is just empty. I feel really lucky and I'm the happiest I've been in my life.'

⇨ The above story is an extract from *21st Century HIV, Personal Accounts of Living With HIV In Modern Britain*, by the Terrence Higgins Trust, and is reprinted with kind permission. Please visit www.tht.org.uk for further information.

Teenagers born with HIV tell of life under society's radar

HIV-positive youngsters who were infected before or at birth reveal their secret lives.

By Amelia Hill

Clive was nine years old when he discovered he was HIV positive. The devastating news that his mother, doctors and support workers had spent years preparing to break to him in the gentlest manner possible, was blurted out by a careless receptionist at his local hospital.

'My mum had bought me to see the doctor because I had earache, and this woman just read it out loud from my notes as she was typing my details into the computer,' says Clive, who celebrated his 18th birthday last week. 'I remember standing there, with my mother's hand around mine, as these feelings of complete confusion and fear washed over me.'

Clive credits the medication given to his mother during her pregnancy for protecting him then from her HIV infection. But, he says, something went catastrophically wrong at the point of delivery, and the infection was passed into his own bloodstream.

After that day at the hospital, however, Clive refused to take medication on his own behalf. 'I suddenly realised that the pills my mum had been giving me every day – that I had thought were sweeties – were medicine,' he says. 'After that day at the hospital, I would lock myself in the bathroom when my mum took them out of the cupboard. Or I'd pretend to swallow them, then throw them away.'

Clive's resistance to taking medication became more deep-rooted as he grew up. 'The medication makes me feel sick – I was sick every time I took it from ten to 13 years old. Other times, I just don't want to remember that side of me. I want to be normal.'

He shrugs sheepishly. 'The last time I stopped taking them was because I broke up with my girlfriend and I had other things on my mind.' Clive takes his pills sometimes, he says, but then stops for months at a time. 'I know I'm killing myself,' he says truthfully, but with studied nonchalance. An exuberant teenager, full of life, he laughs at my shock. Pulling his homburg hat to a jaunty angle, he throws a caricatured 'oh, poor me' puppy dog stare.

But there's nothing funny about Clive's attitude towards his HIV status. A decade of sporadic adherence to his drug regime has stunted the teenager's growth. It has left him close to death three times, and caused him to develop resistance to a number of the drugs that could have almost guaranteed him a long and healthy life. 'I was in hospital again in January,' he says, absently drumming a jazz riff on the table in front of him. 'But my hospital visit before that was the worst: I got pneumonia after stopping taking my meds. My CD4 count [cells that help fight infection] was down so low that I was basically dead.'

There are around 1,200 children like Clive in the UK and Ireland: young people living with perinatally acquired HIV, contracted from their mother in the womb, at the point of delivery or shortly after birth, while being breastfed.

They are a hidden group. Fiercely protected by a medical profession that never expected them to grow from babies into children, much less teenagers, they seek to exist under society's radar, to avoid being branded by the stigma that it attaches to HIV. Over a number of months, however, many of these young people – and HIV-positive women who have had children of their own – told *The Guardian* their stories for the first time.

This group of young people are a singular demographic produced in the few years before medical innovation had caught up with real life. The breakthrough in the 1980s of Haart – highly active antiretroviral therapy – gave these children the chance of a normal lifespan. It also reduced the chance of women with HIV passing the disease on to their babies from around 20–30%, to under 1%. Today, says Pat Tookey, who manages the National Study of HIV in Pregnancy and Childhood (NSHPC), the comprehensive, anonymised surveillance of all obstetric and paediatric HIV in the UK and Ireland, there is 'a vanishingly small chance giving birth to an HIV-positive baby, if medication is taken from the point of conception and all interventions are followed'. 'Thanks to the fact that an HIV test is routinely recommended to all pregnant women during their antenatal care, most with HIV are diagnosed in time to take up interventions,' she says.

But there was a time lag before Haart reduced the likelihood of transmission between mother and baby so dramatically, and when infected babies were still being born. The seismic shift that happened in these few years was that these HIV-positive babies were, for the first time ever, being born into a world where they were able not just to survive, but to thrive.

'In earlier days, most babies with HIV had a short life and our task was to make the quality of that life reasonable,' said Diane Melvin, a consultant clinical psychologist at St Mary's hospital in London. 'We never expected these babies to live. They were certainly not expected to survive adolescence.'

But that is exactly what they are now doing. Of the 1,200 children born with HIV and living in the UK and Ireland today, just 60 are under four years old. Around 400, in contrast, are aged between ten to 14, and another 300 are between 15 and 19. Contrast this to the 1980s, when the first infected babies were born. 'There was no treatment in the early days,' remembers Tookey. 'The babies used to turn up with a symptomatic disease and die.'

For the first time, doctors are daring to hope that children born with HIV can have a normal life expectancy, provided the drugs work and any issues around resistance are solved. 'But this is just an assumption,' warns Tookey, 'We can't be sure of the future because the virus is good at developing resistance to specific drugs, and none of these children have ever lived into middle – or older age.'

Despite medical caution, however, the first cohort of teenagers born with HIV shows every sign of rude health. In what must be the most under-celebrated triumph of modern medicine, in the last two years, the oldest survivors of childhood HIV have grown into young adults.

It is a group that comes in all shapes and sizes: some have problems, some are doing well, some are even starting on their own families. What they all share, however, is the desire to live as normal a life as possible.

'Society forces me to live two lives, one of which – the one where I'm honest about my status – I have to keep completely secret from the other one,' says Clive. 'It angers me that HIV is considered such a dirty thing by so many people. Why are people more sympathetic to those with cancer than those with HIV? It's partly because I have to live this life of shame and secrecy that I find it so hard to take my meds.'

Other young people admit that the stigma of their disease exacerbated their teenage predilection to risk-taking behaviour. 'From the age of five to 17, I had to take 23 tablets a day, and I had to do it in secret because of the ignorance in school and society as a whole,' says Pauline, now 24. 'I got to a point where I had just had enough. I just wanted to block HIV out of my life. I didn't take my meds for a year and a half. Eventually, I was ill for four months, then I lost a stone in three days and couldn't get out of bed. I couldn't breath, my heartbeat was crazy. I thought that was it.'

Pauline alerted a friend, who drove her to hospital, where she spent a week in intensive care. Pauline, who has a young – and uninfected – son of her own, is now a mentor for other HIV-positive children. Asked about the problems faced by children growing with HIV today, she angrily says that, 'from what the young people tell me, the situation around HIV in schools and society in general hasn't improved at all.'

'It doesn't occur to people that you can be born with HIV and live a normal life,' she adds. 'The result is that some of these children go down the same spiral I did and end up in hospital.'

Other teenagers with perinatally acquired HIV, however, refuse to let the disease define them. They take their meds and forge ahead, living confident and strong lives.

Cheerfully tucking into cheesecake while describing her plans for the future, Martha makes a claim that is barely believable. 'If I could live my life again and not be positive, I wouldn't want to,' the 20-year-old announces, giggling at the astonishment – and disbelief – that I fail to wipe quickly enough from my face. 'It sounds weird, I understand that,' she acknowledges. 'But I've achieved more things by being positive than I would have if I had been born negative. It's made me a much more educated person and put some amazing experiences in my path.'

Martha reels off a windfall of opportunities that have come to her, courtesy of her HIV status. 'I have spoken at three international Aids conferences, presented at three Children's HIV Association (Chiva) conferences, met MPs, been a mentor to other young people born with HIV, and have written magazine articles for Positively UK [a peer-led support group for HIV-positive people across the UK].' She pauses for breath. 'If someone offered me a cure, I might take it,' she concedes. 'But not definitely. HIV is a really small part of my life. I have HIV; HIV doesn't have me.'

Even Martha, however, admits that children born with HIV struggle against far greater odds than those growing up with other perinatally acquired diseases. 'I'm angry about the stigma in society that makes me have to lie about my status,' she admits. 'It should be like having a heart disease or high blood pressure. What I want people to know is that we're living normal, healthy lives. We're alive: we were not supposed to be.'

The continuing fear and ignorance about HIV in society, however, continues to make it necessary for young people to lead double lives,

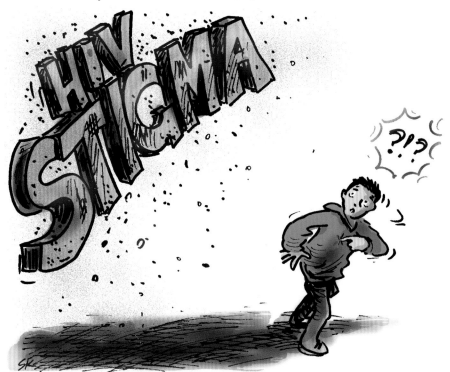

despite the damage that it can do to them.

A recent survey by the National Aids Trust found that one in five adults do not realise the disease can be transmitted through sex without a condom. Fewer than half believe it can be passed by sharing needles or syringes. Around 10% believe it can be transmitted through kissing and spitting – an increase of 100% since 2007.

The stigma that society places on HIV has another, even nastier knock-on effect: it means that children cannot be told of their diagnosis until they are judged to be able to keep it confidential.

The consequence of this is that unlike other childhood diseases, children born with HIV often learn of their diagnosis after they have already absorbed the fear and believed the lies about the disease that swill around society. The trauma can be deep and long-lasting.

In one comprehensive survey, a third of children with perinatally acquired HIV admitted to having considered killing themselves. There can also be a direct impact on a child's lifelong adherence to medication. And this, of course, affects others: statistics show that young people with chronic conditions are more likely to report three or more than four simultaneous risky behaviours than healthy teenagers, including unprotected sex.

But even for those children who adjust well to their status, taking medication is not simple. Nor is hiding it from others: some young people have to take 12 different pills, three times every day.

It is a programme to which they must adhere with relentless precision. 'For treatment to be effective, you need 97% adherence – to within two hours of taking the pill at the same time every day,' says Nimisha Tanna, from Body and Soul, a pioneering charity dedicated to transforming the lives of children, teenagers and families living with, or affected by HIV. 'It is very important,' she adds. 'Otherwise the virus wakes up, mutates and can become permanently resistant to the treatment you're taking.'

Persuading adolescents to take their treatment seriously, however, isn't easy. Just like any other teenager, their health is not their first priority nor organisation their strongest suit. Clinics dedicated to young adults with HIV are springing up to try to help this group.

But, says Dr Caroline Foster, a consultant in adolescent HIV at Imperial College healthcare NHS trust, problems can occur when such facilities are not available and 18-year-olds find themselves ejected from the paediatric care facilities they have attended since they were born into an adult facility, ill-adjusted to their specific needs. 'Adolescent survivors of HIV are a new and challenging population,' says Dr Steven Welch, a consultant paediatrician at Birmingham Heartlands hospital. 'The challenge is that, having got to the stage when we can enable young people to survive with HIV, we can also give them the quality of life to go with it. But this is entirely new territory for us all: paediatric HIV consultants have never had to deal with adolescents, or their parents. And how do we help a young person, for example, who is about to have their first sexual experience but already has a sexually transmitted disease?'

These are challenges the medical profession must surmount, however, because although about 98% of diagnosed pregnant women now take antiretroviral therapy, there are still at least 40 infected babies born in the UK every year.

It happens, says Tookey, for a range of reasons: the mothers sometimes lead chaotic lifestyles or have long-standing undiagnosed infections. Or they get infected during pregnancy, a time when few women would think to use a condom. There are also women who get infected after they have given birth to a healthy baby but while they are still breastfeeding.

'It's probably unrealistic to say we can get that 40 down to zero,' admits Tookey, whose study follows all infants born to women known to be HIV-positive at delivery in the UK or Ireland. 'But we should be able to get it down to ten a year if we can make sure women have every opportunity

to take the test, and if positive, have as much support as they need to enable them to take up the treatment in pregnancy, and avoid breastfeeding.'

That would, of course, be a medical triumph – but those living with HIV are equally concerned that there is a social breakthrough too.

It is because society stigmatises HIV with such 'vicious ignorance', says Pauline, that she dreads the moment she has to tell her young son about her own infection. 'I got pregnant because I was too scared and ashamed to tell the nurse who gave me my 'morning after' pill about my HIV status. I didn't realise that my medication made a difference to how well the contraception would work,' she says. 'I'm hoping that, by the time my son needs to learn about my status, the stigma will have come down and people will be more comfortable talking about HIV. I'm hoping that by then, we won't have to hide any more. That learning of my status will be the same as telling him I've got any other manageable disease.'

She pauses, an elegant young woman with long, immaculately lacquered nails at which she anxiously picks and tugs. 'The fear that my son will judge me for having this disease is something I can't begin to worry about now. Why should he blame me for being born sick? Why should anyone judge me for that?'

Names have been changed

This article was amended on 12 March 2012 to correct one reference that said there are 12,000 children living in the UK and Ireland today who were born with HIV. Elsewhere the article specified the correct figure, 1,200.

11 March 2012

UNAIDS reports more than 50% drop in new HIV infections

UNAIDS reports a more than 50% drop in new HIV infections across 25 countries as countries approach the 1,000-day deadline to achieve global AIDS targets. In addition, the number of people with access to antiretroviral therapy increased by 63% in the last 24 months–AIDS-related deaths fell by more than 25% between 2005 and 2011 globally.

A new World AIDS Day report: *Results*, by the Joint United Nations Programme on HIV/AIDS (UNAIDS), shows that unprecedented acceleration in the AIDS response is producing results for people. The report shows that a more than 50% reduction in the rate of new HIV infections has been achieved across 25 low- and middle-income countries – more than half in Africa, the region most affected by HIV.

In some of the countries which have the highest HIV prevalence

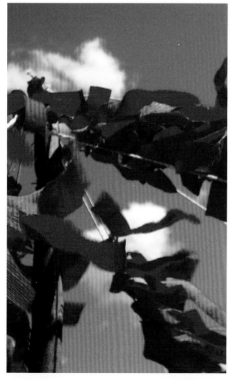

in the world, rates of new HIV infections have been cut dramatically since 2001; by 73% in Malawi, 71% in Botswana, 68% in Namibia, 58% in Zambia, 50% in Zimbabwe and 41% in South Africa and Swaziland.

In addition to welcome results in HIV prevention, sub-Saharan Africa has reduced AIDS-related deaths by one third in the last six years and increased the number of people on antiretroviral treatment by 59% in the last two years alone.

'The pace of progress is quickening – what used to take a decade is now being achieved in 24 months,' said Michel Sidibé, Executive Director of UNAIDS. 'We are scaling up faster and smarter than ever before. It is the proof that with political will and follow through we can reach our shared goals by 2015.'

For example, South Africa increased its scale up of HIV treatment by 75% in the last two years – ensuring 1.7 million people had access to the lifesaving treatment – and new HIV infections have fallen by more than 50,000 in just two years. During this period, South Africa also increased its domestic investments on AIDS to US$1.6 billion, the highest by any low- and middle-income country.

The report also shows that countries are assuming shared responsibility by increasing domestic investments.

More than 81 countries increased domestic investments by 50% between 2001 and 2011. The new results come as the AIDS response is in a 1,000-day push to reach the Millennium Development Goals and the 2015 targets of the UN Political Declaration on HIV/AIDS.

Declining new HIV infections in children

The area where perhaps most progress is being made is in reducing new HIV infections in children. Half of the global reductions in new HIV infections in the last two years have been among newborn children. 'It is becoming evident that achieving zero new HIV infections in children is possible,' said Mr Sidibé. 'I am excited that far fewer babies are being born with HIV. We are moving from despair to hope.'

In the last two years, new HIV infections in children decreased by 24%. In six countries – Burundi, Kenya, Namibia, South Africa, Togo and Zambia – the number of children newly infected with HIV fell by at least 40% between 2009 and 2011.

Fewer AIDS-related deaths

The report shows that antiretroviral therapy has emerged as a powerful force for saving lives. In the last 24 months the numbers of people accessing treatment has increased by 63% globally. In sub-Saharan

Africa, a record 2.3 million people had access to treatment. China has increased the number of people on HIV treatment by nearly 50% in the last year alone.

There were more than half a million fewer deaths in 2011 than in 2005. The largest drops in AIDS-related deaths are being seen in countries where HIV has the strongest grip. South Africa saw 100,000 fewer deaths, Zimbabwe nearly 90,000, Kenya 71,000 and Ethiopia 48,000 than in 2005.

Impressive gains were also made in reducing tuberculosis (TB)-related AIDS deaths in people living with HIV. In the last 24 months, a 13% decrease in TB-related AIDS deaths was observed. This accomplishment is due to record numbers of people with HIV/TB co-infection accessing antiretroviral treatment – a 45% increase. The report recognises the need to do more to reduce TB-related AIDS deaths.

More investments

The report shows that countries are increasing investments in the AIDS response despite a difficult economic climate. The global gap in resources needed annually by 2015 is now at 30%. In 2011, US$16.8 billion was available and the need for 2015 is between US$22–24 billion.

In 2011, for the first time ever, domestic investments from low- and middle-income countries surpassed global giving for HIV. However, international assistance, which has been stable in the past few years, remains a critical lifeline for many countries. In 26 of 33 countries in sub-Saharan Africa, donor support accounts for more than half of HIV investments. The United States accounts for 48% of all international assistance for HIV and together with the Global Fund for AIDS, Tuberculosis and Malaria provide the lion's share of investments in HIV treatment. However, countries must take steps to reduce the high dependency on international assistance for HIV treatment programmes.

1,000 days to go

An estimated 6.8 million people are eligible for treatment and do not have access. UNAIDS also estimates that an additional four million discordant couples (where one partner is living with HIV) would benefit from HIV treatment to protect their partners from HIV infection.

Of the 34 million people living with HIV, about half do not know their HIV status. The report states that if more people knew their status, they could come forward for HIV services.

In addition, there is an urgent need to improve HIV treatment retention rates; reduce the cost of second- and third-line treatment; and explore new ways of expanding and sustaining access to treatment, including domestic production of medicines and innovative financing.

Despite the encouraging progress in stopping new HIV infections, the total number of new HIV infections remains high– 2.5 million in 2011. The report outlines that to reduce new HIV infections globally, combination HIV prevention services need to be brought to scale. For example, scaling up voluntary medical male circumcision has the potential to prevent an estimated one in five new HIV infections in Eastern and Southern Africa by 2025.

The report shows that HIV continues to have a disproportionate impact on sex workers, men who have sex with men and people who inject drugs. HIV prevention and treatment programmes are largely failing to reach these key populations.

'UNAIDS will focus on supporting countries to accelerate access to HIV testing and treatment. Now that we know that rapid and massive scale up is possible, we need to do more to reach key populations with crucial HIV services,' said Mr. Sidibé.

20 November 2012

⇨ The above information is reprinted with kind permission from UNAIDS. Please visit www.unaids.org for further information.

Source: UNAIDS World AIDS Day Report 2012

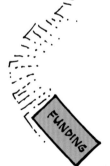

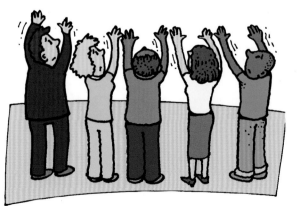

In 2011, an estimated:

- 34 million people globally were living with HIV

- 2.5 million people became newly infected with HIV

- 1.7 million people died from AIDS-related illnesses

The beginning of the end?

Tracking global commitments on AIDS: extracts from the ONE 2012 data report.

The world is off-track for achieving the beginning of the end of AIDS by 2015

There has been mixed progress to date on the three key disease-specific targets tracked in this report: the virtual elimination of mother-to-child transmission; 15 million people on treatment and a reduction in new adult and adolescent HIV infections – all by 2015.

Significant progress has been made on the prevention of mother-to-child transmission, with growing political momentum coalescing around a Global Plan that focuses on 22 high-burden countries. Nearly all of these countries have now developed costed elimination plans, but a significant scale-up of service delivery is necessary in order to increase the rate of progress to reach the virtual elimination target. Access to treatment is the biggest success story, with the global community having achieved unprecedented rates of scale-up, led by investments made

through the US PEPFAR programme and the Global Fund. If current rates of treatment growth can be sustained and moderately scaled up, achieving the target of 15 million people on treatment by 2015 is well within reach. Unfortunately, progress towards the 2015 target of reducing new adolescent and adult HIV infections to 1.1 million is woefully off-track, with more than 2.2 million new infections in 2011.

ONE defines 'the beginning of the end of AIDS' as the point in time at which the number of new HIV infections annually is finally surpassed by the number of people newly added to treatment annually. At current rates of progress, the progression curves for these two indicators will not cross until 2022. To achieve the beginning of the end of AIDS by the end of 2015, the global community will need to add 140,000 people to treatment annually in addition to current rates of treatment growth, and will simultaneously need to double rates of progress on the prevention of new HIV infections.

There is huge variance in donors' responses to the AIDS pandemic

While some donors are stepping up to the plate to make the beginning of the end of AIDS a reality, others are lagging behind, and all could do more.

The United States is far out ahead in terms of financial and political leadership on AIDS globally, providing not just the largest amount of funding but also

setting bold, measurable targets and delivering robust public support for an 'AIDS-free generation'.

The United Kingdom is demonstrating significant leadership on AIDS, and is well positioned to do even more in the coming year. It spends nearly as much ($13.71 versus $14.54) in per capita terms as the US and has outlined a specific AIDS strategy with targets, on which it will report in 2013.

France is the second largest donor to the Global Fund, and AIDS remains consistently high on the agenda for its political leaders. It has yet to develop a clear AIDS strategy with measurable targets, but President Hollande's early public support for the beginning of the end of AIDS is promising.

Germany lags behind in terms of AIDS financing and political support relative to many of its peers, though it has pioneered a number of unique initiatives that support the Global Fund. It has developed a strategy document on AIDS, but that strategy is missing specific targets against which progress will be monitored.

Canada spends far less on AIDS relative to its peers and should scale up both its strategy development and its financing. However, it has made some meaningful contributions. In particular, it has helped to shape global conversations by defining links between the AIDS and maternal and child health policy agendas.

Japan's spending on AIDS fell in 2011 as a result of the catastrophic earthquake and tsunami that hit its shores, leading to budget cuts in the immediate aftermath. However, it has recommitted to its financing for the Global Fund in 2012 as a sign of global solidarity, and should look to rebuild its standing as a significant financial and programmatic contributor to the global AIDS response by following through on its commitments by 2013.

Italy is the clear laggard among the countries analysed. It spent just $5 million on AIDS programmes in 2011,

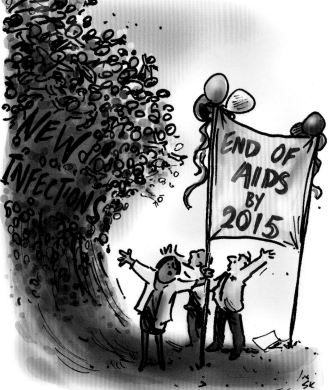

and is the first country to have wholly defaulted on two years' worth of Global Fund pledges.

The European Commission, managing development assistance on behalf of the 27 Member States of the European Union, provides modest funding to the fight against AIDS relative to its other development priorities. However, it remains challenging to track specific AIDS-related outcomes achieved through these investments.

Financing must be increased from current and new sources and must be spent more efficiently

While efforts to improve the cost-effectiveness of AIDS investments are critical, donors must continue to scale up investments in order to achieve the beginning of the end of AIDS goals. UNAIDS estimates that currently there is roughly a $6-billion gap in global AIDS financing annually. Additional resources must continue to flow from donor governments, but resources must also increasingly come from recipient countries in Africa and across the global South. The BRICS countries, as well as private sector and non-governmental partners, have an increasing role to play in providing both funding and expertise.

New investments must also be channelled through national strategies and aligned with investment approaches that improve the targeting and cost efficiency of treatment and prevention resources; doing so will maximise the impact of resources and ensure the strengthening of countries' health systems. Donors must consistently evaluate their bilateral AIDS spending to ensure that the greatest efficiencies are being achieved, and multilateral mechanisms, including UNITAID and the Global Fund, should look for ways to ensure that their resources are being most effectively targeted to maximise disease-specific outcomes.

The global AIDS response is increasingly shaped by developing and emerging economies and non-governmental actors

The financing dynamics for the AIDS pandemic are shifting. While the past two years have seen a levelling off of donor funding, low- and middle-income countries are now providing more than half of total financing to fight the global pandemic. Donor and recipient countries alike are now working in closer partnership, defining targets upfront for how resources are spent for maximum impact and efficiency through national health plans.

African governments are meaningfully stepping up their collective contributions to the fight against AIDS through strategy development and financing. Still, there is much room for growth: approximately 90% of African governments for which we have data are still off-track on reaching their Abuja targets to spend 15% of their national budgets on health, which impedes their ability to scale up domestic resources for AIDS and other health priorities.

Non-traditional partners – including leadership from Brazil, India and China, the private sector and the non-governmental community (including faith-based partners) – are each making new contributions to the fight against AIDS, leveraging their unique skill-sets, relationships and expertise to drive progress where traditional donors are perhaps less well equipped.

A global framework is needed to achieve the beginning of the end of AIDS

Scientific tools are now available to help bend the curve of the AIDS epidemic. What remains missing, however, is a global strategy for how to finance and apply those tools – in conjunction with treatment and care efforts already in place – to accelerate global progress towards the beginning of the end of AIDS. Many donors have outlined important individual efforts, but those efforts are not well coordinated with other donors or with recipient nations, leading to both gaps and duplication of efforts. In addition, although global AIDS targets have been adopted, few donors have outlined what their specific contributions will be towards achieving those targets, leading to a gap in global accountability.

Donors and other stakeholders must come to a global consensus on the imperative of achieving the beginning of the end of AIDS, and should outline specific programmatic and financial shifts that they will undertake to achieve this goal, especially by 2015. In an era of fiscal austerity, these efforts must also include a clear orientation towards maximising results and efficiency gains.

2013 will be a critical test of global commitment

With only three years left to the 2015 goal, 2013 will provide a number of key moments for stakeholders to demonstrate their commitment by following through on or setting new commitments. Most notably, the Global Fund's fourth replenishment meeting offers donors – both traditional and new – the opportunity to reinvest in the Global Fund's critical work to fight AIDS, as well as TB and malaria. A strong show of financial support will position the Global Fund to deliver significant results towards the beginning of the end of AIDS and other critical health targets.

Throughout 2013, global leaders will also be meeting to discuss the future of the Millennium Development Goals beyond 2015. As they discuss and debate a potentially new global development framework, they must not lose sight of the importance of finishing the job on the current set of MDGs – including MDG 6, which focuses on AIDS and other infectious diseases. Leaders should ensure that ongoing discussions incorporate efforts to ensure the achievement of bold health targets already agreed to by global stakeholders.

12 November 2012

⇨ The above information is an extract from the ONE data report *The Beginning of the End?* The extract is reprinted with permission. Please visit www.one.org for further information, or to view the report in full.

Ageing with HIV 'Something we never expected'

30 years ago nobody would have imagined that people living with HIV would live healthy lives through to old age. The advent of effective treatments 15 years ago changed all that and we can now celebrate the fact that people living with HIV are ageing.

But the complications associated with ageing are increasingly being seen as the number one problem in HIV today.

University College Dublin's Dr Paddy Mallon questions whether it's accelerated ageing or accentuated ageing he's seeing among his patients. 'We are probably going to see more cancer and more heart attacks, more fractures, but we have little evidence to suggest this is the case at the moment.'

As we age the cells of our immune system reach a point where they can no longer divide. If you are HIV positive your immune cells have likely been working overdrive to fight HIV so they may reach this end point far sooner, causing inflammation and this contributes to all kinds of age-related diseases. Dr Mallon told BASELINE, 'The HIV immune system bears resemblance to the ageing immune system.'

At 62 years of age Ben Collins has lived with HIV for more than 30 years. He told BASELINE, 'I got tested early along with my work mates. Early and frequent testing was considered 'good manners' and good public health. I got involved as a volunteer. I was a clinical trial subject. I worked in an HIV advocacy organisation. I started treating early. I got LOTS AND LOTS of therapy to deal with stress and my underlying destructive tendencies and self-stigmatisation. I've been in a strong loving relationship for over 20 years. I take my pills regularly. I see my doctor as advised. I am very active.'

Ben does not doubt that HIV puts him at risk of accelerated ageing but says 'it's hard for me to sort what's HIV, what's ageing.'

Rising HIV in the over-50s

HIV is often mistakenly seen as something that predominantly affects younger people. But in the UK HIV is fast rising in the over-50s – in people post-divorce, re-engaging with casual sex, with limited knowledge of HIV or other sexually transmitted infections. Simply put they are people who have a poor understanding of their risk and don't use condoms.

Medics often fail see these people as 'likely candidates' for HIV who have presented to their GP time and time again with symptoms suggestive of HIV but leave without a diagnosis. The fact is that around half of older people diagnosed between 2000 and 2007 acquired HIV at age 50 or older.

New HIV diagnoses more than doubled among the over-50s between 2000 and 2007 in England, Wales and Northern Ireland from 299 cases to 710 cases. In 2010, the figure had topped 850 cases, making up eight per cent of the total new diagnoses.

Being older increases the chance of being diagnosed late. In Ireland around half of the 320 people diagnosed last year were diagnosed late (with a CD4 cell count less than 350), but it rose to 65 per cent among people over 50 years of age.

The increase in the proportion of older people living with HIV requiring complex care will be a challenge to the healthcare system in coming years.

Who is best placed to provide medical services to older people with HIV?

Speaking recently at the British HIV Association Conference in London, Dr Paddy Mallon told delegates, 'We cannot rely on PCTs or GPs to know what is right for our patients. We must retain that power to provide better outcomes for our patients.'

But it's likely that many of us will need to use primary care more and more to manage the complications of living long-term with a chronic disease, whether that's for a statin prescription or blood pressure medication. Many HIV-positive people we spoke to report feeling more confident in doing this than they had in the past, but others

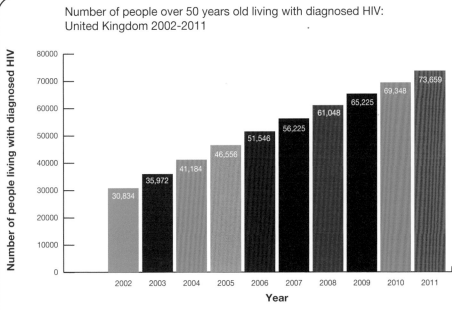

Number of people over 50 years old living with diagnosed HIV: United Kingdom 2002-2011

Number of people living with diagnosed HIV

- 2002: 30,834
- 2003: 35,972
- 2004: 41,184
- 2005: 46,556
- 2006: 51,546
- 2007: 56,225
- 2008: 61,048
- 2009: 65,225
- 2010: 69,348
- 2011: 73,659

Year

Source: HIV in the United Kingdom: 2012 Report, *November 2012 ©Health Protection Agency*

remain reluctant to disclose their status.

More problems sooner?

As people living with HIV age we are likely to be increasingly, some would say disproportionately, affected by chronic illnesses such as heart disease and stroke, high blood pressure, diabetes, kidney disease and liver disease, low bone mineral density as well as cognitive decline and a number of cancers.

Some studies suggest these problems are occurring earlier among people living with HIV. Problems that are usually seen in 60 or 70-year-olds are being seen in 40 or 50-year-olds with HIV.

Michael Snaith, an 'elite controller', told BASELINE, 'I am now 30 years into diagnosis. I tend to say now that I am suffering from age-related problems and not HIV-related problems. Getting old and living with HIV is becoming more of a strain to my health and well-being. Examples, irritable bowel syndrome, long-term depression, pains in my legs and often sleep disorders, just to name a few.'

Around 60 per cent of HIV-positive men in their 40s have osteoporosis or its pre-condition osteopenia – a condition usually not diagnosed in men until their 80s.

People with HIV are also at high risk of chronic lung disease, depression and frailty and there's now some evidence that people with HIV with high blood pressure are at an increased risk of heart attack compared with HIV-negative people.

Dr Mallon told BASELINE, 'the data show that the MI (myocardial infarction, or heart attack) event rate was higher in HIV-positive versus HIV-negative people for a given blood pressure, which suggests that, although rates of hypertension may not be higher in HIV-positive people, the consequences of hypertension in terms of risk of MI may be greater among people with HIV compared with HIV-negative people.'

So why all these complications when we know that HIV medicines are effective? The problem is that despite effective HIV treatment, our bodies remain in an inflammatory state, with our organs facing continuous damage. If you are a smoker or are living with chronic hepatitis B or C too the inflammation appears to get worse.

Depression is a particular problem for older people living with HIV. Speaking at the recent Washington AIDS conference, Stephen Karpiak of the AIDS Community Research Initiative of America said that a 2005 survey of older positive people in New York found that 50 per cent reported depression; 'it's the single most important cause of non-adherence to all medicines, including HIV medication', he told delegates.

Forgetfulness or inability to concentrate can make daily living and importantly, sticking with medicines, a challenge. Amy told BASELINE, 'The fact that we have to work until we are 67 is frightening. How are we supposed to do that, especially if the job is physically demanding and there is rent and bills to pay? It's really worrying me.'

Unemployment among older people has increased rapidly since the beginning of the recession. Since 2008, the number of unemployed people aged 50 to 64 has risen by 53 per cent and the proportion of older people who are unemployed for over a year has risen from 33.2 per cent to 44.5 per cent.

Finding suitable employment can be an even greater challenge if you are living with HIV and have been out of the job market for some time. But returning to work or study can reap other benefits aside from financial – feeling more integrated into a social network; if you're not ready for that step yet, find out if your local HIV organisation is looking for volunteers – it's a great way to meet other people with HIV.

Hope for the future

Last year Italian researchers suggested that a poor diet and illicit drug use are also possible causes of premature ageing, proposing the wider use of anti-inflammatory drugs such as aspirin and statins as possible treatments. The same researchers felt that early HIV treatment in older positive people could help to delay ageing.

Enjoying life and taking good care of yourself; eating well, getting enough sleep, exercising, stopping smoking and reducing alcohol consumption can all contribute to helping you feel well.

Peter Noble, a long-term HIV survivor told us, 'It's a bummer when you've seen friends and lovers die, and you realise you going to be a retired person living with HIV and God forbid we get dementia and forget we have it. Let's just enjoy old age and behave accordingly ... bad.'

We know that HIV treatment works just as well for older people, who often report better treatment adherence, so do keep taking the tablets.

'Disease mongering' is not helpful according to Dr Mallon; 'we'll know more as people living with HIV age.' Ben Collins is clear that it's important to stay informed; 'If you've got a problem or a question get help. Denial is silly. Get involved.'

This article was commissioned and sponsored by Janssen-Cilag Limited (Janssen). The views expressed are those of the author. Janssen is one of the world's leading research-based pharmaceutical companies with a heritage of innovation in HIV. The company seeks to be an innovative and socially responsible participant in the response to HIV/ AIDS in order to save and improve the lives of those living with HIV and prevent the further spread of the virus.

16 November 2012

⇨ The above information is reprinted with kind permission from BASELINE. Please visit www.baseline-hiv.co.uk for further information.

© *Fieldhouse Consulting Ltd, 2012*

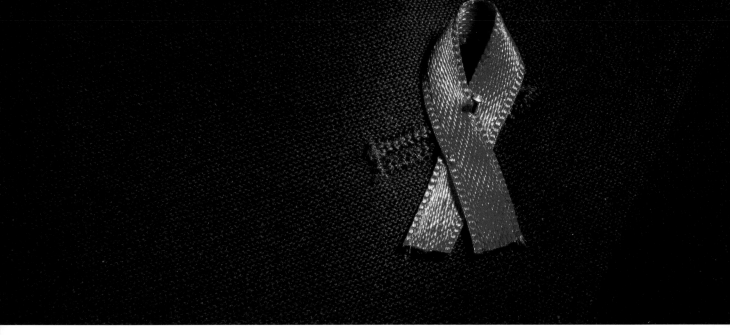

First patient 'cured' of HIV?

By Cara Acred

Timothy Ray Brown, from San Francisco, had been living with HIV for over a decade when, in 2006, he was diagnosed with leukemia. Brown moved to Germany in 1993 and was treated for his leukemia at a clinic in Berlin where, after unsuccessful chemotherapy, doctors gave him a bone marrow transplant from a donor who had a genetic resistance to the HIV virus.

Brown's case was first reported to the media in 2008. At this point, 20 months after the bone marrow transplant, he seemed to be completely free of both the leukemia and the HIV.

Professor Rodolf Tauber, from the Charite clinic, said: 'This is an interesting case for research. But to promise to millions of people infected with HIV that there is hope of a cure would not be right.'

HIV is estimated to have infected 33 million people worldwide, but only one in 1,000 Europeans and Americans have a resistance to HIV and could act as donors.

Professor Andrew Sewell of the University of Cardiff said 'The problem is most people with HIV live in sub-Saharan Africa and this is hugely expensive, you have to find a matched donor, and it's a pretty severe and painful operation. So it's going to be an option for very few people.'

In 2012, at a symposium on gene therapy at Washington University, Brown told The Associated Press that his body is 'proof of the concept that HIV can be cured.' Despite claims that he still has traces of HIV in his body, Brown said that any remaining virus was dead and that he believed he would be 'the first of many people who will be cured of the AIDS virus'.

Brown is now working with the Washington-based World AIDS Institute to raise money that will fund research to find a cure for the virus.

15 March 2013

⇨ The above article was written by Cara Acred, on behalf of Independence Educational Publishers.

Researchers step up efforts to find an HIV cure

By Keith Alcorn

'Berlin Patient' Timothy Brown has 'inspired the field'

Scientists launched a road map for research into an HIV cure ahead of the 19th International AIDS Conference (AIDS 2012) in Washington DC, promising international collaboration and calling for more funding to be devoted to research that can eventually deliver a course of treatment that will, at the minimum, allow people with HIV to remain off medication for life even it can't eradicate HIV from the body.

The 'Towards an HIV Cure' declaration marks a substantial shift in the scientific consensus regarding the feasibility of HIV cure research. Over the past four years funding has begun to flow towards small intensive studies that will contribute towards cure research. Worldwide attention has been grabbed by the case of the 'Berlin Patient', Timothy Brown, who was pronounced cured of HIV infection after a gruelling course of chemotherapy, immunosuppressive treatment and a bone marrow transplant from a donor with a rare genetic resistance to HIV infection.

'I don't think anyone would want to go through what he went through to get that cure, but it has inspired the field,' Dr Steven Deeks of the University of California San Francisco, told a press conference launching the International AIDS Society's cure research strategy prior to a pre-conference symposium, Towards an HIV Cure.

Support for a comprehensive effort to cure HIV infection is also driven by the mounting long-term cost of HIV treatment. By 2015, US$24 billion will be required to provide treatment for 15 million people; at least 35 million people are estimated to be infected with HIV, and eventually all will be eligible for HIV treatment. A cure which can be feasibly delivered at a large scale in countries with weak health systems, and which is affordable, will begin to look more and more attractive to major international donors as treatment costs continue to rise.

What do scientists mean by an HIV cure?

An HIV cure requires either the clearance of HIV from every cell in the body, or the establishment of a sufficiently strong immune response to keep HIV in check when medication is stopped. The difficulty of achieving eradication of the virus lies in the fact that HIV can remain latent within CD4+ T-cells and some other immune system cells for many years, and cannot be detected by the immune system. It is only when those cells are activated by an external stimulus that they begin to produce HIV. These cells form a 'reservoir' of latent virus that could cause viral rebound as soon as antiretroviral treatment is stopped. It would take the activation of only a few infected cells to cause viral rebound; the reservoir of latently infected cells probably comprises thousands of cells.

The case of Timothy Brown is the only example of an HIV cure that has been scientifically validated, but even this case raises questions about what a cure means. Scientists talk about two possible outcomes from cure research: eradication, where the virus is cleared from the body, and a 'functional cure', where tiny amounts of virus may persist, but the virus remains controlled without medication.

The HIV field had thought that the case of the 'Berlin Patient' represented the first example of HIV eradication, but recent data presented at the International Workshop on HIV & Hepatitis Virus Drug Resistance and Curative Strategies in Sitges, Spain, in June, indicated that some laboratories which had tested samples of plasma and tissue from the 'Berlin Patient' Timothy Brown, had been able to detect very low levels of HIV DNA or RNA several years after the interventions. This suggests that HIV has not been completely eradicated from this patient's body. Yet, not all laboratories were able to detect HIV, and the finding remains controversial.

Professor Sharon Lewin of the Alfred Hospital, Melbourne, commented: 'My gut feeling is that it's not real. My take on it is that the DNA and RNA samples were looked at by labs that are very experienced in this work, and in a sub-set of these laboratories there was some evidence of RNA and DNA, which may or may not be contamination. There may be contamination in the best-run labs. He certainly doesn't have virus that is infectious or that has rebounded to a detectable level. If it's real, we still have a fantastic example of a functional cure.'

Dr Steve Deeks said that the findings, which his 'gut feeling' tells him to be evidence of real virus, suggest three take-home messages. Firstly, more sensitive tests are needed for measurement in HIV eradication studies. Secondly, immune responses may be the most important indicators of the achievement of a functional cure, even where evidence of virus persists; Timothy Brown's antibody levels continue to decline, suggesting that not enough HIV is being produced to stimulate immune responses. Finally, all the clinical signs suggest that the patient is doing well in the absence of antiretroviral therapy, again suggesting that any persisting low-level HIV infection that might exist is causing no physical harm.

Indeed, given all the sites and cell types that HIV may infect, a functional cure may be more feasible – and may be perfectly satisfactory for people with HIV, depending on how that affects their everyday lives.

'I asked patients in Asia recently what they wanted and they didn't say a cure, they said "a treatment I can stop"' Professor Francoise Barré-Sinoussi told the press conference.

Research conducted among people living with HIV in The Netherlands, on the other hand, suggests that when presented with different attributes of a potential curative course of treatment, people want a treatment that removes long-term uncertainty about health and side-effects, ends stigmatisation and ends the risk that they will infect partners. People living with HIV rate the psychosocial benefits of a cure very highly when asked to rank a range of possible health and psychosocial benefits, Fred Verdult told the Towards an HIV Cure symposium.

A cure, functional or otherwise, and an end to AIDS will also depend on reaching people who have HIV: those who know it and those who don't. 'What would a cure have to look like to access that group of people who are currently not either diagnosed or on treatment?' asked Steven Deeks.

Path to a cure

Views differ on what might be the most productive approach towards curing HIV infection, and researchers emphasise that there is still a great deal of ground to be covered. Tony Fauci, director of the US National Institute of Allergy and Infectious Diseases, described the 'false start' of the mid-1990s, when some researchers assumed that viral suppression on HAART, and the absence of new rounds of infection or evolving HIV DNA, meant that replication had been halted and that eradication was only a question of waiting a few years for all the HIV-infected cells to die a natural death. Robert Siliciano and others soon demonstrated that HIV was infecting cells that might persist for years, and that estimates of HIV eradication after a few years of HAART were wildly optimistic.

All researchers agree that a cure, functional or otherwise, will depend on

a combination of approaches. Where they disagree is on the ingredients of the cocktail.

A cure for every patient will need to start with a prolonged period of antiretroviral therapy to reduce HIV to undetectable levels. This period of treatment itself could be important in determining the success of subsequent drug therapies. Will attempts to purge the HIV reservoir be more successful in people who began treatment very soon after infection? A French cohort has produced tantalising data suggesting that some people treated in acute infection can stop treatment and go for very long periods – an average of 72 months so far – without experiencing viral rebound. What is it about these people that prevents viral rebound? Is it the time they started treatment, their genes, or just random chance?

Scientists are also interested to learn whether any form of intensified antiretroviral drug regimen could shrink the pool of latently infected cells, making them easier to purge later. So far, studies have shown little or no impact of regimens drawing on the maximum number of drug classes on the size of the reservoir of latently infected cells, but further studies are planned, using more sensitive measurement techniques, to see whether five-drug combinations that target every possible step in the viral lifecycle have more effect.

Studies are also underway or planned to determine the extent to which the viral reservoirs can be emptied by using a range of drugs that will activate latently infected cells so that they can be identified and killed by the immune system, or self-destruct.

Sharon Lewin of the Alfred Hospital, Melbourne, described the range of studies already taking place using compounds called HDAC inhibitors, which stimulate latently infected cells to begin producing HIV. A number of experimental studies with HDAC inhibitors are already underway, most notably with vorinostat (SAHA). This drug is already approved for the treatment of cutaneous lymphoma, and is currently undergoing phase II tests for a range of other malignancies, so its short-term toxicities are well

characterised. In vitro toxicity studies suggest a potential long-term risk of malignancy, but at this point no human studies have reported an increased risk of malignancy. Sharon Lewin's team is studying the effect of 14 days of vorinostat (SAHA) in 20 patients with fully suppressed viral load, and will measure the effect of vorinostat on cell-associated HIV RNA to determine the effect of the drug on HIV latency.

"We don't want someone saying it's going to take X million dollars and X years ... because we don't want to over-promise what we can't deliver"

Professor David Margolis at the University of North Carolina is conducting a similar experimental study, measuring the effect of a sequence of single doses of vorinostat on virus production in up to 20 volunteers with fully suppressed viral load. Steven Deeks at the University of California San Francisco is testing the anti-alcohol agent disulfiram, which also activates latently infected cells. Preliminary data presented at CROI in 2012 showed that this agent stimulated HIV RNA production in a sub-set of chronically infected patients who received the drug.

In addition to these agents, there are six or seven known targets for therapies that could disrupt HIV latency, and in collaboration with Merck, Professor Margolis's research group has identified 83 compounds with differing mechanisms of action that are being tested for their potential as disruptors of latency. Two other companies, Gilead and Janssen-Tibotec, are also engaged in major screening programmes to identify agents that could contribute towards cure research.

Ultimately a number of different agents may need to be used in combination, said Warner Greene of the Gladstone Institute, San Francisco, in order to target the different points in the transcription pathway that govern the integration and latency of HIV in cells.

Activating agents might also need to be used in combination with a therapeutic vaccine to stimulate the immune system to clear the activated cells, because researchers are still uncertain how long the activated cells will continue to produce virus once activated, and whether cells which are not fully activated are nevertheless capable of producing virus that will go to infect other cells. (Activation is a cycle rather than an on/off process.)

Researchers are also investigating gene therapy approaches that can gradually establish a pool of HIV-resistant CD4 cells. This approach is already being studied in people with HIV, but more work is needed to refine the technique and determine whether this approach can contribute towards an HIV cure.

The long and winding road

Questions of cost and scaleability will loom ever larger as researchers make progress towards a cure, but at this stage leading players are stressing the need for realistic expectations about how long this research will take.

'I can't tell you how long it will take or how much it will cost, but now we are collaborating, it will take a considerably shorter time,' said Rowena Johnston of AmFAR, who is leading the organisation's efforts to fund innovative cure research as a means of kick-starting a larger cure research effort.

How much it will cost and how long it will take to get there are matters of pure conjecture at the moment, and advocates and researchers are reluctant to commit themselves on either question. 'The reason we don't want someone saying it's going to take X million dollars and X years is because we don't want to over-promise what we can't deliver. But if we put in more money we will get there sooner,' said Johnston.

The research effort will also need to overcome the scepticism of a field that has seen several major breakthroughs fail to materialise.

Tony Fauci pointed out how many times the 'you can't do it' school have been proved wrong in HIV research, starting with antiretroviral therapy, all the way through to efforts to deliver treatment in the developing world, to the recent PrEP studies. HIV research requires great feats of discovery, but it also requires the discovery of an approach to a scaleable cure to mobilise the resources, he told researchers.

22 July 2012

⇨ The above information is reprinted with kind permission from NAM Publications. Please visit www.aidsmap.com for further information.

Campaigners demand more HIV testing

Patient campaigners warned that people are still involved in risk-taking behaviour because they do not think they will get HIV.

Barriers to testing for the infection have also led to late detection and have prevented people from benefiting from early treatment, it was claimed.

Dr Jack Lambert, infectious disease consultant at the Mater Hospital, warned a late diagnosis could lead to the rapid onset of AIDS.

'We have to continue challenging the stigma that still surrounds HIV in Ireland in order to effect change,' said Dr Lambert. 'The public needs to know that by avoiding early HIV testing, you put yourself at risk of rapid disease progression – possibly leading to AIDS.'

A total 6,287 people in Ireland have been diagnosed with HIV since the early 1980s. Latest figures from the Health Protection Surveillance Centre showed 30% of people living with HIV are unaware of their infection.

While the overall diagnosis rate decreased by 3% in 2011, more than half of the 320 people who tested positive presented late with the illness. And 27% of the 85 women newly diagnosed were pregnant.

The highest proportion of new cases was among men who have sex with men (42.5%), while a third were heterosexual men and women, and 5% were injecting drug users. Three mother to child cases were diagnosed.

The figures were released ahead of Irish AIDS Day – on Friday June 15 – when a 'Don't Guess, Get Tested' campaign will be launched by Open Heart House, the Sexual Health Centre, AIDS West, Dublin AIDS Alliance and the Red Ribbon Project. Deirdre Seery, chair of HIV Service Network, said healthcare professionals should challenge the stigma surrounding HIV and testing.

'Late presentation of HIV is a significant problem in Ireland and despite attempts to encourage earlier testing for HIV, this situation is of serious concern,' Ms Seery said. 'In Ireland, as with other countries, there are still many people involved in risk-taking behaviour and because they don't perceive themselves as being at risk of HIV they don't avail of HIV testing.'

11 June 2012

⇨ The above article originally appeared on BelfastTelegraph. co.uk and is reprinted with permission. Please visit www. belfasttelegraph.co.uk for further information.

It's time to allow home testing kits for HIV in the UK

By Rachel Carrell

A GP told me last week he couldn't remember the last time a woman had come to see him for a pregnancy test. Home pregnancy tests are now so accurate, there's no need to see a doctor.

It's strange now to think that the medical profession was quite unsure about home pregnancy tests when they were first launched. In 1978, just as the first home pregnancy tests were hitting the market, one concerned doctor from prestigious hospital Johns Hopkins told the *New York Times*, 'Pregnancy is a very emotional event and people don't [use home tests] as well as they might. They have a hard time following even relatively simple instructions.'

In the years that followed, women all over the world decided that even if home tests were a bit less accurate than their doctor would be, they also had big advantages. Convenience. Privacy. Anonymity. The chance to cry in your own loo.

Nowadays, of course, home pregnancy tests are as easy to get as toothbrushes. But it seems we haven't learned the broader lesson about letting people make their own decisions about how they get tested.

When it comes to HIV status, we still don't trust people to test at home. In the UK, while it's legal to offer HIV home sampling (in which you post off the sample to a laboratory), full HIV home tests – the kind where you find out the result in your bathroom – have been prohibited since 1992.

It's high time that ban was lifted.

Back in 1992, positive HIV status was virtually a life sentence. Thankfully, that's no longer the case. HIV treatment has improved so much that people with HIV live for decades. You can now get life insurance as an HIV-positive person. There's even emerging evidence that people with HIV who make it to the age of 60 may have longer-than-average life expectancy.

Despite that, this week India's National AIDS Control Organisation announced it won't be lifting its own ban on HIV home tests. An official explained, 'We don't want people to self-test and then commit suicide or self-harm because they are HIV positive.'

I'd say learning you're HIV positive is roughly the same level of 'life changing' as learning you're pregnant.

The real public health risk comes not from suicide, but from people who don't realise they have HIV passing it on to others. In the UK, a quarter of those with HIV don't know they have the virus. But a recent survey of people with HIV found that over a third would have been diagnosed earlier if home-testing kits were available.

We should make home tests available in the UK. We should encourage high-risk people to use them often. We'd need to regulate them properly, be upfront about the tests' accuracy, and make sure they come with details of where to get further advice and support. In lifting the home-testing ban we would be following the lead of the United States, where the FDA approved an HIV home-testing kit for the first time in July this year.

The broader principle in all of this is also important. It didn't end with pregnancy tests and it doesn't end with HIV tests. It's this: what the medical establishment values isn't always the end of the story. Things that patients value, like convenience and privacy, can be just as important – or even more important, when it makes the difference between people accessing and not accessing healthcare at all. The difference between an HIV test that's quite accurate and one that's very accurate might be important. But the difference between either of those things and an at-risk person not getting tested at all is much bigger.

We need to give patients a variety of options, supported by clear, evidence-based information and advice, and allow them to make their own decisions. It's all part of healthcare's retail revolution.

26 November 2012

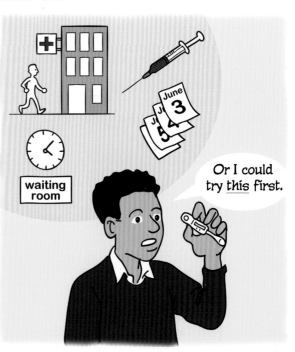

'As close to an HIV cure as we've seen': breakthrough hailed as radical treatment works on baby born HIV positive in Atlanta

US team gave child stronger, faster dose of antiretroviral drugs straight after birth.

By Kunal Dutta

Scientists appeared a step closer to conquering the AIDS virus after US doctors confirmed they had cured an infant born with HIV through a course of antiretroviral drugs, the first time this has ever been recorded.

Doctors in Atlanta said a two-and-a-half-year-old child from Mississippi was born HIV positive and received a three-drug infusion within 30 hours of its birth, a stronger and far swifter dose than normally administered.

"US doctors confirmed they had cured an infant born with HIV through a course of antiretroviral drugs"

Last night scientists confirmed that the child, whose identity has not been disclosed, has since been off medication for HIV for over a year, is believed no longer to be infectious.

"Not all traces of the virus have been eradicated"

Last night scientists were pouring over the findings, unveiled at the Conference on Retroviruses and Opportunistic Infections in Atlanta. 'You could call this about as close to a cure, if not a cure, that we've seen,' said Dr Anthony Fauci of the National Institutes of Health. Much of the success of treatment is believed to be down to the swiftness and intensity of the antiretroviral dosage that was so potent. Usually a child is given a course of one drug.

While the findings are encouraging, scientists warned they are not the definitive cure for HIV. It is thought to have been the speed and intensity of the action that knocked out HIV in the baby's blood before it could form hideouts in the body. But not all traces of the virus have been eradicated. Dr Deborah Persaud of Johns Hopkins Children's Center, who led the investigation, said that the child was in effect 'functionally cured', meaning in long-term remission even if all traces of the virus haven't been completely eradicated.

The treatment would not work in older children or adults as the virus will have already infected cells. The number of babies born with HIV in developed countries has fallen dramatically with the advent of better drugs and prevention. Typically, women with HIV are given antiretroviral drugs during pregnancy to minimise the virus in their blood. Their babies go on courses of drugs, too, to reduce their risk of infection further. The strategy can stop around 98% of HIV transmission from mother to child. About 300,000 children were born with HIV in 2011. In the US such births are very rare as HIV testing and treatment have long been part of prenatal care. 'We can't promise to cure babies who are infected. We can promise to prevent the vast majority of transmissions if the mums are tested during every pregnancy,' said Dr Hannah Gay, of the University of Mississippi.

The only other person considered cured of the AIDS virus underwent a bone marrow transplant from

"There may be different cures for different populations of HIV-infected people"

a donor naturally resistant to HIV. Timothy Ray Brown of San Francisco has not needed HIV medications in the five years since that transplant. The Mississippi case shows 'There may be different cures for different populations of HIV-infected people,' said Dr Rowena Johnston of amFAR, the Foundation for AIDS Research. That group funded Persaud's team to explore possible cases of paediatric cures. It also suggests that scientists should look back at other children who've been treated since shortly after birth, including some reports of possible cures in the late 1990s that were dismissed, said Dr Steven Deeks of the University of California, San Francisco. 'This will likely inspire the field, make people more optimistic that this is possible,' he said.

4 March 2013

⇨ The above article originally appeared in *The Independent*, and is reprinted with permission. Please visit www.independent.co.uk for further information.

Baby cured of HIV: was this a premature release?

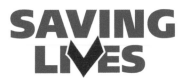

By Dr Steve Taylor, Medical Director of Saving Lives and HIV Consultant.

www.savinglivesuk.com

On Monday 4 March, the world awoke to a media storm: news was buzzing around the world that a Mississippi baby had been cured of HIV.

We were soon bombarded with a flurry of media reports about how this case was set to change the HIV treatment paradigm, prevent babies from being infected, and, to quote the principal author of the study, Dr Deborah Persaud, 'transform our current treatment practices in newborns worldwide'.

I'm currently in Atlanta in the USA, where this research was presented at the Conference for Retroviruses and Opportunistic Infections. The news stations here are already asking if this means that children who are infected at birth can stop their drugs. They're asking when the cure will be available, and patients have even been calling their paediatricians at this meeting, raising the question of whether their child could also be cured!

To which I say: STOP. Back up. Rewind.

To quote a famous professor of HIV pharmacology: 'We need more data.' We need to take stock, get the facts right, and allow for scrutiny of the case by the scientific community.

There are many questions to be asked of the case. For instance, was the baby truly infected in the first place? From reviewing the data presented at the conference, it certainly seems possible. But how established was this infection? Had it established itself in so-called long-lived memory T cells?

Furthermore, when was the actual point of infection? This is not clear. Could it have been just prior to delivery? If so, it is possible that by serendipity the doctors intervened with drugs just as the virus was trying to become established.

It's imperative, then, that we attempt to understand when exactly this baby was infected. Was it just before birth, or several months before birth? The longer the period of time, the more interesting the case becomes.

However, if the intervention simply aborted the establishment of infection then Dr Persaud's results are less exciting.

If drugs were introduced very shortly after infection, the treatment may have actually acted as 'post-exposure prophylaxis' – a strategy already used by HIV doctors to try and avoid establishment of infection.

Think of a fire which has just caught alight, but has yet really to take hold. Pouring a bucket of water on it at this point may kill the fire dead. Was there actually a flame, or the presence of detectable virus, in this case? Yes, of course. But this bucket of water may not have worked had you allowed the 'fire' to become properly established.

The case being described by many as a 'cure' may in fact be like this bucket of water – effective, but only because it was delivered so early.

Taking the fire analogy further, after we have put out the flames we may still see the residues it left behind. It might even reignite at a later point in time. The Mississippi baby has been off antiretroviral drug treatment [ARVs] for less than a year – there are currently no flames, but we are waiting to see if the embers are truly burned out.

Currently, and beyond this headline case, we have no way to completely put out the fire of HIV once it has caught hold. Our current ARV treatments, then, are the firemen who keep the flames of HIV at bay. As long as they are there, you can begin to rebuild the house – a fact born out by the fact that hundreds of thousands of our patients have been on totally suppressive regimens for up to 20 years.

Currently, it is a truth that, if you stop therapy, the virus inevitably rebounds when you do – usually within two weeks. Admittedly, there are a very few rare cases where the virus may simply smoulder away at very low levels for many years (so-called 'post-treatment controllers').

All of these considerations and unanswered questions mean that we have a long way to go yet before we fully understand this case. We must fully explore the baby's immune make-up. What about the characteristics of the mother's virus, which was curiously low for someone not on treatment? There are so many questions before we should really call this a cure.

Other than the potential of Dr Persaud's research to stimulate further investigations, then, what is the best thing that can come of all this media frenzy?

The great hope is that this moment represents the greatest mass HIV awareness campaign since the Don't Die of Ignorance 'tombstone' campaign of the 1980s. Rarely does HIV make such headlines, and we have a real chance to educate people whilst their interest is piqued.

We must tell people that the story of HIV is very different now, and we must take this opportunity to communicate new messages through the media whose attention we currently have – messages which can correct people's out-dated misconceptions.

Let's talk about testing, and the importance of early diagnosis.

Let's talk about effective drugs, which

when prescribed early enough can help a patient live a long and full live.

Let's talk about condoms and prevention.

Let's tackle stigma.

Today there is no reason for any baby to be become HIV positive, if the mother is tested and diagnosed early in pregnancy – and if she and the baby have access to effective treatments which can prevent transmission. Sadly, 590,000 babies every year are still born HIV positive in the developing world: an unnecessary tragedy.

We can do something about that right now, with the tools we have – If we increase testing and make it more regular and consistent. In the UK, 95% of women take the HIV tests during pregnancy. And with effective treatment the chance of the baby being born positive is less than 0.5%. We should be aiming for the same success all over the world

Above and beyond a media storm about a supposed 'cure', there are good news stories we can make happen today.

Is the 'cure' story exciting? Yes. Is it scientifically plausible? Yes. Will it stimulate more research? Almost certainly. But it is extremely premature to hail it as a cure that will translate into routine clinical care any time soon. We need much more data.

So if you or your child are HIV positive, then please ... don't stop taking your tablets. And if you have had unprotected sex, take the test. Condoms, education, testing, and access to treatment are our real weapons against HIV, and we need to learn to use these correctly if we want to make a real impact today.

7 March 2013

⇨ The above article appeared on TheHuffingtonPost.co.uk and is reprinted with permission from AOL (UK). Please visit www. huffingtonpost.co.uk for further information.

Reports of HIV 'cure' are premature

Analysis by Bazian. Edited by NHS Choices.

Global news coverage has been dominated by the potentially groundbreaking news that a child born with HIV appears to have been 'cured' of the infection.

The Guardian reports that US doctors have made medical history with a 'first functional cure' of an unnamed two-year-old girl born infected with HIV and 'who now needs no medication'. BBC News quotes researcher Dr Deborah Persaud, who presented the news to a medical conference, as saying, 'This is a proof of concept that HIV can be potentially curable in infants.'

The researchers report that the baby was started on antiretroviral (anti-HIV) treatment at two days of age and continued on this to 18 months. By one month old, HIV could no longer be detected in the baby's blood using standard laboratory tests, and the virus continued to be undetectable up to 26 months of age. However, highly sensitive laboratory tests could still detect the presence of HIV at very low levels.

This means that scientists have not found a complete cure for HIV. However, as *The Guardian* clarifies, they have found a 'functional cure', in which the girl is still infected, but currently requires no treatment. This means the disease is less likely to progress in the girl, potentially giving her a good life expectancy.

It is not yet possible to say whether this child's viral levels will remain low, or whether she will need further antiretroviral therapy.

These findings therefore do not mean that a complete cure for HIV has been discovered.

We are still a long way short of a 'cure' for HIV.

The potential outcome of treatment for the baby girl in the current US case is unclear. She is likely to need further blood tests as she grows up, to keep a check on the levels of HIV in her blood. Hopefully, she will continue to grow healthily into adulthood with the virus at undetectable levels. However, it is possible that she may need further ART if her viral levels begin to rise again.

It is impossible to say how or why this particular child has achieved a 'functional cure'. It could be the fact that she had very early treatment with ART, or it could be due to the biology of this individual child.

The next step for researchers is to see whether the ART regime used for this child causes a similar outcome for other high-risk newborns.

It is currently uncertain whether the information contained in this case report will lead to any advances in the treatment of older children or adults with HIV. ART is prescribed on an individual basis according to clinical tests, response and adverse effects. Anyone taking ART should continue to take the treatment as prescribed by their specialist.

The findings do not mean that a new complete cure for HIV has been found.

However, if the results can be replicated in other newborns, it may offer the hope of reducing the number of cases of infant HIV in the developing world.

4 March 2013

⇨ The above information is reprinted with kind permission from NHS Choices. Please visit www.nhs.uk for further information.

Key facts

⇨ In 2010, sexual transmission accounted for about 19 in 20 new confirmed cases of HIV in the UK. (page 1)

⇨ The number of new HIV diagnoses in the UK peaked at 8,000 in 2006 and dropped to 6,660 in 2010. The total number of people living with HIV in the UK in 2010 was 91,500. (page 2)

⇨ The estimated number of people living with HIV (both diagnoses and undiagnosed) in the UK in 2011, infected through injecting drugs, was 2,300. (page 2)

⇨ In 2011, the overall prevalence of HIV in the UK was 1.5 per cent of the population, with the highest rates reported among men who have sex with men (MSM). (page 5)

⇨ In 2011, 6,280 people were newly diagnosed with HIV in the UK, a 21% decline from the peak in new diagnoses in 2005. (page 5)

⇨ Less than 1% of infants born to women diagnosed with HIV prior to delivery acquired perinatal infection in 2010/2011. (page 5)

⇨ In 2011, 70% of all sexually transmitted infection clinic attendees received an HIV test, with the highest coverage among MSM (83%). (page 5)

⇨ Worldwide, 2.5 million people became newly infected with HIV in 2011. (page 6)

⇨ 25 countries have seen a 50% or greater drop in HIV infections since 2001. (page 6)

⇨ TB-related deaths in people living with HIV have fallen by 25% since 2004. (page 6)

⇨ In 2011, there were almost 2 million AIDS related deaths. (page 6)

⇨ In low- and middle-income countries with available data, 91% of total spending on HIV programmes for sex workers comes from international sources, as does 92% of spending on HIV programmes for MSM and 92% of spending on HIV programmes for people who inject drugs. (page 7)

⇨ In 2010, the Health Protection Agency estimated that one in 20 gay men in the UK live with HIV. (page 8)

⇨ More than two in five (44 per cent) gay and bisexual men have never discussed STIs with a healthcare professional. (page 9)

⇨ A quarter of young people responding to the Sex Education Forum survey (2011) said that they had not learnt about HIV and AIDS in school. A further 11% could not remember if they had learnt anything. (page 10)

⇨ The overall proportion of people living with HIV in the UK was estimated to be 0.15%, or one in 650. The proportion of men living with HIV in the UK was estimated to be 0.20%, or one in 500, while the proportion of women living with HIV in the UK was estimated to be 0.09% or one in 1,000. (page 14)

⇨ Of those receiving HIV care in 2011, 36,355 were exposed through sex between a man and a woman, 31,825 were exposed through sex between men, 1,636 were exposed from injecting drug use, 1,488 were exposed from mother-to-child trans, mission and 533 were exposed from blood/receiving blood products. (page 14)

⇨ In the US in 2001, 17% of people with HIV were over 50. Now, that figure stands at 39% and by 2017 it will be half. (page 18)

⇨ In the UK and Ireland, there are around 1,200 children living with HIV that they contracted from their mothers in the womb, at the point of delivery or shortly after birth. (page 23)

⇨ Half of older people, diagnosed between 2000 and 2007, acquired HIV at age 50 or older. (page 30)

⇨ Around 60 per cent of HIV-positive men in their 40s have osteoporosis or its pre-condition osteopenia. (page 31)

AIDS

Acquired Immune Deficiency Syndrome. AIDS is a potentially fatal illness. It develops at the most advanced stage of HIV.

Antiretroviral therapy

Drugs that suppress the amount of HIV virus in the body. Antiretrovirals (ARVs) help people with HIV to live relatively healthy lives for a long time, although they do not cure the condition.

'Berlin Patient'

Timothy Ray Brown, from San Francisco, was nicknamed the 'Berlin Patient' after being treated in Berlin in 2006. He and his doctor claim that Brown is the first person to be cured of HIV, thanks to a blood stem cell transplant using a donor with a rare gene mutation that provides natural resistance to HIV.

Criminalisation

Making something illegal. Deliberately infecting another person with HIV, or knowingly putting them at risk of infection, is now a criminal offense.

Discrimination

Treating someone differently/less favourably because they are different. The misconceptions and negative attitudes surrounding HIV and AIDS can lead to discrimination in many different circumstances.

Epidemic

Widespread occurrence of an infectious disease.

Ethnicity

Ethnic origin.

HIV

Human Immunodeficiency. A virus passed-on through certain bodily fluids such as infected blood, genital fluids, breast milk and semen. It cannot be passed through kissing or touching. HIV attacks the cells of the immune system, making it hard for the body to fight infections. Immediately after contracting HIV, a person may experience flu-like symptoms which will then disappear. At later stages of infection, symptoms include fatigue, weight loss, sores in the mouth and pneumonia. HIV can, eventually, progress to AIDS.

Immune system

The immune system is made up of cells, tissue and organs that protect the body from viruses and infections. The HIV virus attacks the immune system and prevents the body from protecting itself.

Prejudice

Referring to prejudgement – forming an opinion before you are fully aware of the facts.

Sexually transmitted disease

A disease or infection that is transmitted through the exchange of bodily fluids such as semen or genital fluids.

Stigma

A negative reaction associated with a particular circumstance. Being HIV positive has a 'stigma' attached – it often causes others to behave negatively because they are wary of contracting the virus themselves, through touching or close contact, and can invite preconceptions about a person's sexuality or sexual promiscuity.

Tuberculosis (TB)

A bacterial infection spread through inhaling tiny droplets from the coughs or sneezes of an infected person. This is a serious condition but can be cured with proper treatment. Symptoms include a persistent cough, weight loss, night sweats and high temperature.

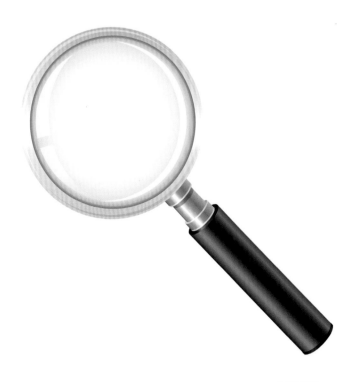

Assignments

1. Design a leaflet that will be displayed at your local GP's office, explaining AIDS and HIV, include information about how they are contracted and what treatment is available. You should also provide details of how and where people can be tested.

2. Read the article *HIV in the United Kingdom* on page 5 and write a summary for your school newspaper.

3. Research the history of AIDS and HIV. Are there any important developments that have been missed out of the *History of an epidemic* timeline on page 7? Reproduce the timeline, adding anything from your own research that you think is important.

4. Read the article *Why are African people and gay men more at risk of HIV?* on page 8. Choose one of these groups – African people or gay men – and research the HIV statistics for that group. Create a flyer that summarises the key statistics for your chosen group.

5. Imagine that you are an Agony Aunt/Uncle. Write a response to the following letter:

Dear Agony Aunt/Uncle,

I am a 26-year-old man and have been in a relationship with my current girlfriend for six months. In the past, I have had unprotected sex with both men and women, and I'm worried that I might have contracted an STD. I know I should get tested, but I'm scared that my girlfriend will leave me if I have caught something bad.

6. In small groups, discuss what you have been taught about AIDS and HIV at school. Create a detailed plan for a lesson that will teach pupils of your age-group about these illnesses. Think carefully about what should be included and consider how you will make the lesson interesting and memorable.

7. Read the article *Criminalisation of HIV transmission* on page 11. Using the Internet, research cases in which someone has intentionally infected another person with the HIV virus. Make some notes on the cases you find and feedback to your class.

8. Design a website that will offer help and advice to those who have tested positive for HIV. Produce samples of your home page and at least three other pages.

9. In small groups, discuss the stigma surrounding AIDS and HIV. Make a list of the misconceptions and negative attitudes that people with AIDS and HIV have to confront, and think about the consequences of these attitudes.

10. Watch the film *Philadelphia* (1993), starring Tom Hanks. Write a 500-700 word essay answering the following question: 'How does the film Philadelphia (1993) address the social stigma surrounding AIDS and HIV?'

11. Look at the map *AIDS and HIV: the regional picture* on page 17. Choose a country on a different continent from your own and research the prevalence of AIDS and HIV in that country. You should also research treatment options and awareness. Make some notes on your findings and feedback to your class.

12. Imagine that you have recently been diagnosed with HIV. Write a blog post expressing your feelings and thoughts. How do you feel right now? What challenges do you think you will have to overcome? What does the future look like? How will your life change?

13. Research the Terrence Higgins Trust and create a presentation explaining what they do. You could include case studies from people who have been helped by the Trust, examples of their research, etc.

14. Choose an illustration from this book and think about how it complements the article it accompanies. What is the artist trying to portray? Are they successful?

15. As a class, discuss whether home-testing kits for HIV are a good idea. Do you think they would encourage people to get tested?

16. Create a campaign that will raise awareness of AIDS and HIV amongst people your age. What kind of campaign would be most successful? Television, radio, web or posters? Produce a campaign plan and include sample designs, scripts or storyboards.

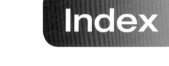

Index

Acknowledgements

The publisher is grateful for permission to reproduce the following material.

While every care has been taken to trace and acknowledge copyright, the publisher tenders its apology for any accidental infringement or where copyright has proved untraceable. The publisher would be pleased to come to a suitable arrangement in any such case with the rightful owner.

Chapter 1: AIDS & HIV

AIDS and HIV © 2013, Egton Medical Information Systems Limited, HIV in the United Kingdom © Health Protection Agency, Global facts: World AIDS day 2012 © UNAIDS Global Fact Sheet 'World AIDS Day 2012', History of an epidemic © 2013 AIDSARK, Why are African people and gay men more at risk of HIV? © Lloydspharmacy Online Doctor 2013, Gay and bisexual men's health © Stonewall 2011, Young people's experiences of HIV and AIDS education © The Sex Education Forum, Criminalisation of HIV transmission © NAM publications 2013, Coping with a positive HIV test © NHS Choices 2012.

Chapter 2: Living with AIDS & HIV

People living with HIV in the UK © National Aids Trust 2013, What is stigma? © 2010 eSchooltoday, Stigma and discrimination © NAM Publications 2013, Study identifies issues affecting the quality of life of patients living with HIV © NAM Publications 2013, HIV survivors: alive but facing poverty, loneliness and prejudice © Guardian News and Media Limited, 21st Century HIV © Terrance Higgins Trust 2013, Teenagers born with HIV tell of life under society's radar © Guardian News and Media Limited.

Chapter 3: Developments

UNAIDS reports more than 50% drop in new HIV infections © UNAIDS World AIDS Day Report 2012, The beginning of the end? © ONE 2012, Ageing with HIV 'Something we never expected' © Fieldhouse Consulting Ltd, 2012, First patient 'cured' of HIV? © Cara Acred/Independence Educational Publishers Ltd., Researchers step up efforts to find an HIV cure © NAM Publications 2013, Campaigners demand more HIV testing © Belfasttelegraph.co.uk, It's time to allow home testing kits for HIV in the UK © 2013 AOL (UK) Limited, 'As close to a cure as we've seen': breakthrough hailed as radical treatment works on baby born HIV positive in Atlanta © independent.co.uk, Baby cured of HIV: was this a premature release? © 2013 AOL (UK) Limited, Reports of HIV 'cure' are premature © NHS Choices 2013.

Illustrations:

Pages 5, 27: Don Hatcher; pages 10, 36: Angelo Madrid; pages 24, 28: Simon Kneebone.

Images:

Cover and pages i & 32 © Instamatic, pages 13 & 14 © Moon Ape Media, page 16 © David Dallaqua, page 18 © Sergio Roberto Bichara, page 20 © Leroy Salstad.

Additional acknowledgements:

Editorial on behalf of Independence Educational Publishers by Cara Acred.

With thanks to the Independence team: Mary Chapman, Sandra Dennis, Christina Hughes, Jackie Staines and Jan Sunderland.

Cara Acred

Cambridge

May 2013